Springer Series on Nursing Management and Leadership

Joyce J. Fitzpatrick, RN, PhD, MBA, FAAN, Series Editor

Advisory Board: Pamela Cipriano, PhD, RN, FAAN; Harriet Feldman, PhD, RN, FAAN; Greer Glazer, RN, PhD, CNP, FAAN; Daniel J. Pesut, PhD, APRN, BC, FAAN

Joyce J. Fitzpatrick, RN, MBA, PhD, FAAN, FNAP, is the Elizabeth Brooks Ford Professor of Nursing at the Frances Payne Bolton School of Nursing, Case Western Reserve University, where she teaches courses on management and health policy for advanced practice nurses. She also is a Visiting Scholar at Mount Sinai Medical Center in New York. Dr. Fitzpatrick has held many leadership and management positions in nursing education and professional organizations. Her MBA degree, received from Case Western Reserve University in 1992, was focused on health care management.

Beverly Ann Glasgow, RN, BSN, MS, MSN, is a Family Nurse Practitioner (FNP) at the Family Medicine Clinic of Oxford in Mississippi. She received a BS and Masters degree in Health Care Administration from the University of Mississippi, a BSN from Union University, and a MSN from the University of Tennessee. She is a doctoral candidate in the Case Western Reserve University Bolton School of Nursing Doctor of Nursing Program for advanced practice nurses. She has an extensive background in both nursing education and nursing practice. She has been Director of a Primary Care Clinic for 6 years and a FNP for 2 years. Her doctoral research is focused on FNP 's adherence to clinical practice guidelines. Her future goal is to establish a rural health care center in Mississippi and obtain certification as Emergency Nurse Practitioner to work in the initial telemedicine rural emergency rooms in Mississippi.

Jane N.Young, RN, MSN, CRNP, is President of Family Health Care in Boise, Idaho. She received undergraduate degrees from both Boise State University and Montana State University, and a MSN degree from the University of Portland. She completed the Nurse Practitioner certificate program at the University of Washington and is certified as a Pediatric, Adult, and Family Nurse Practitioner. She currently is a doctoral candidate in the Case Western Reserve University Bolton School of Nursing Doctor of Nursing Program for advanced practice nurses. She was among the first nurse practitioners in the northwest, and currently owns and manages her own practice, Family Health Care. She has over 25 years in practice as an advanced practice nurse. Her doctoral research is focused on trust in the nurse practitioner patient relationship. Her future goal is to continue to serve her community and her patients through an integrated mind/body approach to health care.

Managing Your Practice

A Guide for
Advanced Practice Nurses

Joyce J. Fitzpatrick, PhD, MBA, RN, FAAN
Ann Glasgow, MSHCA, MSN, FNP
Jane N. Young, CRNP, MSN
Editors

 Springer Publishing Company

Springer Publishing Company, Inc.
536 Broadway
New York, NY 10012-3955

Acquisitions Editor: Ruth Chasek
Production Editor: Matt Fenton
Cover design by Joanne Honigman

03 04 05 06 07 / 5 4 3 2 1

Library of Congress Cataloging-in-Publication Data

Managing your practice : a guide for advanced practice nurses / Joyce J. Fitzpatrick, Ann Glasgow, Jane N. Young, editors
    p. ; cm.
Includes bibliographical references and index.
ISBN 0-8261-1934-4
    1. Nursing—Practice. 2. Nursing services—Administration. 3. Nursing services—Business management. I. Fitzpatrick, Joyce J., 1944– II. Glasgow, Ann. III. Young, Jane N.
    [DNLM: 1. Nurse Practitioners. 2. Practice Management. 3. Nursing—organization & administration. WY 128 M2667 2003]
RT86.7.M36 2003
362.1′73′068—dc21

2003045425

Printed in the United States of America by Sheridan Press.

Contents

Contributors

Mary K. Bailey, RN, FNP, ND
Assistant Professor
Mennonite College of Nursing
Illinois State University
Normal, IL

Susan Comstock, MS, RN, CNM
Assistant Professor of Nursing
California State University,
    Sacramento
Sacramento, California

Anita England, BS, RN, MSN, ND
Emergency Department Nurse
Marymount Hospital
Garfield Heights, Ohio

Trish Goudie, RN, MSN, CNM
Dean, College of Nursing
Montana State University-Northern
Havre, Montana

Elizabeth Bodie Gross, RN, FNP, MS, MBA, CCM
Elder Link
Barrington, Illinois

Barbara M. Henrichon, RN, FNP, NDc
Emergency Room Nurse Practitioner
Park Ridge Hospital
Rochester, New York

Barbra J. Keller, BSN, RN, MSNc, FNP
Operating Room Nurse
Regional Medical Center
Alamosa, Colorado

Barbara L. Kennedy, MA, MN, RN, FNP-C
Lecturer
California State University –
    Dominguez Hills
Carson, California

Joni L. Thanavaro, RN, MSN, ANP, ND
Associate Professor of Nursing
St. Louis Community College at
    Meramec
St. Louis, Missouri

Jeani C. Thomas, MSN, FNP-C
Director of Mobile Health
Our Lady of Bellefonte Hospital
St. Christopher Drive
Ashland, Kentucky

Cheryl W. Thompson, MSN, RN, APRN, BC
Assistant Professor of Nursing
York College of Pennsylvania
York, PA

Andrea Wolf, MSN, CRNP
Family Nurse Practitioner
Family Practice Associates
Lancaster, PA
Coordinator, FNP Program
Widener University
Harrisburg, PA

Preface

Currently there are more than 250,000 Advanced Practice Nurses (APNs). These include nurse practitioners (NPs), certified nurse midwives (CNMs), clinical nurse specialists (CNS), and nurse anesthetists. Most of these APNs are certified in their specialty practice area by a national credentialing organization. The American Nurses Credentialing Center (ANCC) certifies the majority of NPs and CNS advanced practice nurses. Both the midwives' and the nurse anesthetists' organizations have their own certifying arm.

APNs practice in a wide range of settings, including health care organizations of every type. More recently, there has been a movement of APNs into professional practice arrangements that require knowledge of basic business principles and skills in organizing, leading and managing a business, whether the APN is in independent practice or in a practice arrangement with colleagues in other disciplines. In fact, it is often the case that APNs are in collaborative practice with physicians. Whether the practice is solo or collaborative, knowledge and skills in business are most advantageous.

This book is designed as a basic reference for the APN. It is intended to answer the initial questions related to establishing and maintaining an APN practice. Each of the topics was selected because of its relevance to the common goal of designing a practice. Some of the topics are relevant across the practice settings in which APNs work, including strategic planning, credentialing and continuing education, negotiation, leadership, information management, quality management, and ethical issues. Some of the topics are more specific to APN practice that is designed using a business model of care delivery. APNs who are starting their own businesses must concern themselves with financing, risk management and legal issues for maintaining a business and a professional practice. In addition to the topics included in each chapter, the appendices included here provide a wide range of resources for the APN. There are important lists included, such as the certifying boards for specific practice areas, the state licensing agencies, and a summary of the state positions on prescriptive authority for nurse practitioners. Also included in the appendices are sample patient survey questions that can be a part of the marketing strategy, a leadership self-assessment questionnaire for the APN, and an ethical decision-making worksheet. Three sample business plans, each for a different kind of practice that might be established by APNs, are provided as an additional resource.

Each of the chapter contributors is an APN; many of them have been in practice for more than 20 years, others have more recently developed their practices. Many of the contributors learned the principles of business management through their own and others' experiences. Previously there has not been one source for obtaining this basic information. It is our hope that this will serve as a resource for APNs who are currently in practice and those contemplating practice.

—Joyce J. Fitzpatrick

Managing Your APN Practice: The Basics

1

Jane Young
Ann Glasgow
Trish Goudie
Joyce J. Fitzpatrick

What is a mission statement?

A mission statement is a statement of purpose. It explains why your practice exists. A mission statement provides excitement, clarity, and, especially, inspiration. It is used to help initiate, evaluate, and define your activities. In the form of a directive, your mission statement needs to be understandable in lay terms and embedded in your memory so that it can be easily recalled. Keep your mission statement at hand: You will reference it frequently.

When developing your mission statement, reflect on your nursing philosophy and your practice. Carefully answer the following three questions: What available population needs does your practice serve? What is your practice doing to address and satisfy those needs? What are the principles and beliefs guiding your work? Your mission statement should reflect your vision. Write your sentences in the present tense, for instance, "I am" (not "I will be" or "I was"). When speaking, use the first person (I, me, or my). Be bold. A mission statement is not a solution, but rather a means to achieve your goals. Make sure your goals meet the SMART criteria: Specific, Measurable, Achievable, Relevant, and Timely.

Which is first: writing the mission statement or creating the vision?

The process of developing your vision and mission is interactive. Think about what you envisioned when you first conceptualized your practice. Engage a close friend in recounting the details that started you on your quest of the perfect practice. Who was involved in your vision? What was happening? What were the results? Ask yourself the following questions: "Where do I see myself in 3 years? What about in 5 years? If everything succeeds better than predicted, what will my practice look like? What goals or purposes will have been met? Is my vision achievable? Does it spur me on to explore new arenas?" Your vision and mission will shape the details of your business plan.

Why is a business plan necessary?

A business plan is one of the first requirements for an APN developing a practice. A well-thought-out business plan with financial projections over the first 5 years often is required to gain financial support. When defining the services, you will need to address both immediate and long-term goals. The time and effort you spend making the care you offer better for the patient and different from competitive practices will help you in the long run. It is worth the investment of time required to develop a comprehensive business plan.

As a practicing APN, how will a business plan help you?

A good business plan produces a choice of future opportunities. The financial projections will assist you with making decisions about various opportunities. The plan will guide your decisions so that they are based on an articulate set of rules. These rules are well-defined boundaries that establish priorities and short- and long-term strategies for action. A business plan is the crux of decision making in a viable practice.

What is included in a business plan?

A carefully developed business plan is a competent guide through finance, staffing, operations, and evaluation. The basic components of a business plan are as follows:

- **Executive summary.**   An executive summary is a concise description of your practice. It outlines services, products, markets, competition, and finances. Your summary serves as an introduction to the practice for readers such as investors and possible partners. An executive summary beginning with your mission statement and ending with a list of 1- and 5-year goals is the most effective.
- **Table of contents.**   All components of the business plan should be included here.
- **A basic description of the APN practice.**   The description begins with a vision supported with personal goals and a mission statement for the practice. An organizational chart defines the number and kind of employees, and their relationships. Key managers and employees are included in the job descriptions. Physical facilities, including location and layout (rent, lease, or buy), are also described. Financing should be projected in detail.
- **Products and services.**   Practice services should be based on an estimation of the population served. This description of services defines the practice. Identify the market share (the percent of the health-seeking population) you plan to serve. Describe your standards for the quality and quantity of the proposed services. Be conservative in your timeline but include the order and timing of services to be offered.
- **Operations.**   The operations portion of the business plan describes the location of the practice and details the personnel required for meeting practice goals and the scope of services. Legal aspects include state laws and rules governing a license to practice. Hours of operation and call coverage are established in the operations portion of the plan. This section also lists the

equipment required to support the services you offer, noting those you choose to subcontract, such as dictation, janitorial, laboratory, or other.

- **Marketing.**   Search the current state of the market to find the particular niche your practice will fill among health care services already in the community. Developing a marketing strategy is a very important component of business planning.
- **Competition.**   Find out what other practices offer the type of care you plan to provide. Count the number of practices like yours within a 3-mile radius, and describe the market and services they offer. Friends will volunteer information about their appointments with your competitors, or you can phone the competitors as a patient and schedule an appointment yourself. Knowing your competition is the first step to getting a competitive edge.
- **Risks.**   Know your risks. Identify the obstacles to your practice such as competition, finances, and marketing before they happen. With a well-defined business plan, many of the problems can be identified and resolved with minimal risks.
- **Finances.**   Structure your practice and finances conservatively, realistically estimating the start-up costs. Include the projected costs of operation for each time period or, expressed another way, the number of dollars needed to run your practice per month. Integrate the expected monthly profit and projected income.
- **Milestones.**   Anticipate major events along the timeline for achieving your business goals. Investors and staff should understand every hurdle and success you anticipate happening in the first year of practice. Milestones are your "To Do" list for your practice.

How do you determine which vision is your real vision?

Before developing an APN business plan, be able to answer the following questions:

- What are your vision and mission?
- What is the heart of your vision? What is the most important theme?

- Does your mission support your vision?
- What is your mission's method for accomplishing a vision for your practice?
- How effectively does your vision describe your goals?
- Is your vision clearly stated?
- Does your mission cover the first 5 years of operation? Lay out your mission statement on a 5-year schedule. As you realize progress, ask yourself, "What still stands in the way of achievement?"

How do you define your practice organization?

As you organize your practice, choose an organizational structure that fits the goals you want to achieve. During the process of establishing your mission and goals, ask at the state level about business regulations pertaining to your practice. It will be necessary to register your practice as a business with the secretary of state and the state board of nursing or medicine (whichever has the authority to define the scope of services your practice will offer) before opening the door for business. It is your responsibility to register your practice and conduct periodic evaluations to determine if the practice is operating consistently within the stated vision.

How do you develop your marketing plan?

A marketing strategy describes and measures the patient population your practice expects to serve. It seeks to determine the number of patients, the size of your practice, and the need for services. Will your practice include referrals to or from specialists? Will you welcome walk-ins or will patients be required to have appointments, or both? What are your office hours and will they meet patient needs? What major types of patients exist in the specified area (retired individuals, young families, and similar categories)? Is the number of patients seasonal? Recording the increases and decreases of 5-year evaluations of the markets will help you predict future possibilities for services.

Once the market is identified, determine what percentage of the population you hope to serve each consecutive year you are in practice. How many people do you plan on seeing each day? How soon can you expect to break even?

As you develop your market plan, how will you evaluate your practice in terms of quality? When will the first patient surveys, evaluating baseline satisfaction with your practice and its services, be completed? When will the next evaluation begin? How will you evaluate your financial performance? Does the income-expense statement and balance sheet meet your expectations? Periodically reevaluate the market trends (including the population, economics, and health care system) for your area; integrate the results with the patient-satisfaction surveys as you review marketing strategies. Will your marketing strategy include setting charges? Consider teaching community groups as markets for your services (e.g., an 8-week class on menopause, a 6-week seminar on couple's communication, or a brief lecture discussing birth control). Have you anticipated seeking local charity support, or giving complimentary health-related talks and chairing community presentations? Are you contemplating participation in local nurse practitioner groups to encourage referrals? Define ways in which your marketing strategy might change as your goals are achieved.

How do you develop your financial plan?

Forecasting planned income means determining resources before making spending choices. It is possible to return to a plan and adjust it as the practice develops. Assume you are the only provider. During your total work hours each week, how many patients will you see? What income will that number of people generate? For example, scheduling eight 1/2-hour appointments and sixteen 15-minute appointments on each of the 5 days in a week may be a reasonable beginning.

What if market research tells you the local going rate of a 15-minute patient office appointment is $65? Your goal is to charge less than the average, so you estimate your charges at $50 per 15-minute appointment and $100 per 30-minute appointment. This estimation totals $1,600 per day if every appointment is filled and kept. According to your expectations, your scheduling calendar will be at least half filled during the first year and fully filled by the end of the third year. For Year 1, this results in $800 per day, or $16,800 every month (there are approximately 21 working days in a month), in charges for your direct services.

Compare area laboratory charges with charges from the laboratory you have chosen. Say that you add a 20% markup amounting to an average of $2.50 per test and an additional drawing fee to the lab cost. You estimate an average of four lab tests per visit and one fourth of the patients who visit have laboratory work done. If you see 12 patients a day in Year 1 and one fourth (3 patients) of those require blood work, the estimated drawing fee is $5 each ($15) for a total of 3 patients per day in Year 1. Per month, your drawing fees will average $315 ($15 × 21 working days). Your net income is $30 per day (Year 1) on your markup of the laboratory tests (3 patients × 4 tests each × $2.50 per test markup). Per month, your laboratory markup will average $630 (21 average working days in a month). For a monthly total, add to the $16,800 the number of office visits a month, $315 a month for laboratory drawing fees, and $630 a month for the laboratory test markup. This total allows a possible initial total budget of $17,745 per month. If you are practicing in an area with a lot of managed care, it is reasonable to plan on collecting 87% of your total charges. Theoretically, you can count on $15,438.15 per month in your operating budget. In an effort to add to it, you teach community groups. Their word of mouth offers marketing with no increased expense, and you can collect your fees ahead of time, allowing for 100% collection. This example describes the initial thought process that you will need. The first year will likely seem slow, so adjust your thinking. The numbers will always be estimations, yet, as experience increases, these estimations will approach reality.

Decide how many staff members are necessary to generate the income desired. Make every effort to secure qualified staff. In the meantime, budget for staff turnover until your practice is established.

To determine how much space is needed for the practice to operate, calculate how many exam rooms are needed to keep patient flow progressing at the level required to produce the projected income. What is the approximate size of each exam room, the waiting room, the front office, file space (current and future storage), supply storage, laboratory and nursing stations, staff offices, hallways, cleaning and coat closets, and restrooms? Do they meet the Americans with Disability Act (ADA) requirements? You will need a locked drug cabinet and space to store pharmaceutical samples. To determine an affordable total square footage, estimate your practice's income, staff expense, and additional anticipated expenses. The advice of local merchants (suppliers) and peers already in practice is invaluable. Once operating costs and staff salaries are met and reserves are established, the remaining money helps define your space.

You need to include other space-related expenses, such as janitorial services, utilities, and available parking. Are you charged rent or rent plus other fees for the practice space? If the space is leased, is it triple net (utilities and taxes are included in the quoted lease payment) or are you responsible for utilities on top of your lease payment? Have you established a reserve fund for space maintenance (e.g., carpet cleaning, painting, and light bulbs)? Is business and personal property insurance a lease requirement? Include staff- and provider-related costs in the budget, for example, salaries, benefits, time off (sick and vacation pay), insurance (health and/or liability), professional licensure expenses, unexpected accidents, professional organization expenses, books, and journals.

Daily operational expenses include office equipment (copiers, phones, fax, computers, a server, printers, beepers, and answering machines), office supplies, files, cabinets for charts, chart shelves, patient books, and shelves. These expenses also include medical equipment (otoscopes, ophthalmoscopes, sphygmomanometers, and stethoscopes), gowns/drapes, exam tables, stools, lights, a refrigerator/freezer for immunizations, height/weight scales, and medical supplies. You will also have to purchase equipment shelves, toys, waiting room furniture and supplies (magazines, books, and patient information materials), and janitorial supplies.

Once you have identified the operating costs, list the start-up costs. Consider the following items: In each instance, what is the initial cost of leasing, renting, or buying practice space? What will the cost be in 5 or 10 years? Is adjacent space available for expansion and parking? How accessible is your practice space to the population you expect to serve? Are you required to pay renovation and/or remodeling costs to meet

ADA requirements or practice needs? If so, how much and how often? All these questions enter into the original planning. What staff is essential? Which types of insurance are required, and what accounting and legal services do you need? When is the first tax deposit due? When must you meet the first payroll? What are the costs (time and dollars) of advertising for staff?

Itemize the indispensable equipment (office and medical) needed to operate your practice daily. What furniture and supplies (medical, office, and janitorial) will be necessary the first month? What safety and training devices (e.g., fire extinguishers, emergency medications, and Occupational Safety and Health Administration [OSHA] plans and kits) are mandatory? Is your replacement fund adequate?

What is your timeline?

The following nine steps are offered as a guide to plan an orderly timeline for your practice. Assign a beginning and end date for each step, and include the time needed for accomplishment:

1. Success depends on a preliminary study and review of your initial business plan. This results in a written, workable plan of action.
2. Secure a business license. Prepare financial documents (income-expense statement and balance sheet). Choose a bank and investors. Select your accountant and attorney, and share your business plan with them. Begin the process of selecting a board of advisors if you choose to have one.
3. Begin a marketing plan. Check deadlines and costs for phone-book and newspaper advertising. Note speaking options and area club meeting times.
4. Hire qualified staff. Take the necessary time to read the job description with applicants, orienting them with a clear vision of the practice. Be specific when discussing and delineating each staff member's role in the practice. Tell applicants what is expected of them each day. Pay attention to their dress, personal language, and behavior. Make sure they understand. (Do not

assume.) When hiring, there must be no doubt about your expectations. Have them repeat the description and explanations. Make your staff selections carefully.

5. Diligently search for an appropriate, affordable practice space. Negotiate civilly, sincerely, and fearlessly. Establish a written agreement and provide required remodeling and expected completion dates that are realistic. Include itemized costs in this written agreement. Once this is accomplished, locate and purchase start-up office medical equipment, supplies, and used/new furnishings.

6. Round up your support and take a moment to appreciate your accomplishments before looking ahead with an even clearer focus on your objective of improved patient health care.

7. Open the door and welcome patients.

8. After 6 months, as you analyze the practice finances with your accountant, begin to incorporate the review results into your thinking and make the necessary adjustments.

9. One year following opening day, complete your continuous quality improvement (CQI) program, for example, computing, accounting, billing, your economic statement, patient concerns, practice strengths, health care in general, the national and local market, and population trends.

What does it take to manage a practice?

Management is often considered a special kind of leadership. Managers coordinate and integrate resources through planning, organizing, directing, and controlling to accomplish specific institutional goals and objectives. Nursing management uses these processes to carry out the goals and objectives of excellence in nursing care.

How do management principles work in an APN practice?

In an established clinical practice, the APN is the nurse manager. The management process is similar to the nursing process and consists of four steps: planning, organizing, directing, and controlling. The first step is to gather information (assessing) and then decide which objective(s) needs to be accomplished (diagnosing). Nurse managers then make a plan (planning) before organizing and directing the plan (implementing). Because nurse managers have authority, either through an organization of which they are a part or in their role as independent practitioners, they are also responsible for the process by which these steps are carried out. How do nurse managers determine which goals and objectives are relevant? Whether the APNs are independent or part of an organization, the established mission statement drives the practice. Goals are developed that reflect that mission. Strategic planning describes the process of creating a mission statement and goal setting.

Planning is the process of determining the short- and long-term goals and tasks necessary to accomplish those goals. Planning requires that the manager first gather information in order to make decisions of what to do. Plans can be broad or general, making them easier to change as the need arises. (Specific and detailed plans are less flexible for modification.) Information gathering is vital to the process. Planning errors lead to misinformation, faulty assumptions, and faulty reasoning.

Organizing is the process of gathering all the resources (human and material) necessary to carry out a plan. Skipping this step or only partially completing it leads to a waste of time and resources, and can be expensive.

Directing is the talent of coordinating personnel to carry out the tasks necessary to achieve specific objectives. This involves *motivation*, the process of moving others to action. What motivates one person does not necessarily motivate another. Managers should focus on motivators that work toward self-actualization, such as the following:

- Achievement
- Recognition
- Responsibility
- Advancement
- Growth

The previous internal motivators are greater than external factors, such as salary and scheduling—although there is a certain amount of motivation from those factors, too. Internal and external motivations provide the means for maintaining a satisfying, productive workplace.

Nurse managers with enthusiasm, sensitivity, and creativity, who understand the complexities of nursing practice, will experience the greatest success in getting their team to accomplish their highest goals.

Controlling, an integral part of the management process, means ensuring that tasks and/or strategies are appropriately performed. Managers provide feedback to their team members as they attain objectives, and adjustments are made accordingly. Controlling is a form of evaluating ongoing activities (hopefully resulting in high standards and goal achievement).

What qualities make an APN a good manager?

Successful APN managers are problem solvers. They need a great deal of persistence, intelligence, critical-thinking skills, tolerance, and the ability to not personalize other people's criticisms. These traits, which are so necessary for earning an advanced graduate degree, certification, and licensure, also serve the APN manager. Managers perform the following specific tasks:

- Develop peer relationships.
- Carry out negotiations.
- Motivate subordinates.
- Resolve conflicts.
- Establish information networks and disseminate information.
- Make decisions in ambiguous situations.
- Allocate resources.

How do APNs plan for change?

Planned change occurs when a well-thought-out and deliberate effort is made to make something happen. It involves the application of knowledge and leadership skills of problem solving, decision making, and interpersonal and communication skills. The APN becomes the change agent, which is the person responsible for determining avenues to progressively achieve the change desired. It is up to this person to lead others through the stages of change. A person with an entrepreneurial spirit can inspire others to become integral parts of the change process and can value their input to assist in a better transition to the desired outcome.

Change should be implemented only for good reasons. Individuals need a balance between stability and change within the workplace to be productive. The following are good reasons for change:

- Change to solve some problem.
- Change to provide better care.
- Change to make work procedures more efficient so that time will not be wasted on relatively unimportant tasks.
- Change to reduce unnecessary workload.

Since change disrupts the homeostasis of a group, measures that minimize stress are important. Change agents need to consider four things to support the ability of others to cope with the change:

- Their flexibility to change
- Their evaluation of the immediate situation
- The anticipated consequences of the change
- Their perceptions of what they have to lose or gain

The most critical factor contributing to the resistance encountered with change is a lack of trust between the employee and supervisor or organization. Trust is based on predictability and capability. Those involved want a secure, comfortable environment. They also want a clear understanding that the organization is capable of making a successful change. Therefore, it is wise to include those involved in a change when planning for a change.

What are the leadership roles and management functions in planned change?

A change planned by an APN can be greatly influenced with the following roles and functions:

- Leadership roles
  ➢ Be visionary in changes needed within the practice and health care system.

➤ Choose a risk taker as the change agent.
➤ Have the flexibility to adapt goals during change.
➤ Anticipate and adapt to resistance to change.
➤ Act as a role model to others to stimulate growth by change.
➤ Communicate support to followers during change.
➤ Create alternatives to resolve problems.
➤ Be sensitive to the timing of change.
• Management functions
➤ Forecast the needs within the organization.
➤ Recognize the need for change and the options available to implement change.
➤ Accurately assess barriers to change.
➤ Identify and implement strategies to minimize resistance to change.
➤ Solicit input from those involved in the change and provide them with adequate information during the transition.
➤ Support and reinforce the efforts of others during the change process.
➤ Identify and implement strategies to modify resistive behavior.

What are the stages of change APNs must know to facilitate planned change?

In order to facilitate the change process, APNs need to consider the following three phases:

• Unfreezing
➤ Gather data.
➤ Accurately diagnose the problem.
➤ Decide if change is needed.
➤ Make others aware of the need for change.
• Movement
➤ Develop a plan.
➤ Set goals and objectives.
➤ Identify areas of support and resistance.
➤ Include everyone who will be affected by the change in its planning.

- ➢ Set target dates.
- ➢ Develop appropriate strategies.
- ➢ Implement the change.
- ➢ Be available to support others and offer encouragement during the change.
- ➢ Use strategies for overcoming resistance to the change.
- ➢ Evaluate the change.
- ➢ Modify the change, if necessary.
- Refreezing
  - ➢ Support those involved so that the change remains.

How do APNs manage change?

APNs are involved in managing change in several different ways. The following three phases are important in managing the change process:

- Envision change.
  - ➢ Development of a future vision
  - ➢ Desired future—the big picture
  - ➢ Shared interests and goals with others
- Enable change.
  - ➢ Strategic choices to enact the change
  - ➢ Choices made by the change agent of plans that will affect others
- Implement change.
  - ➢ The "how" of the change process
  - ➢ Making it happen

APNs can use the following guide for managing successful planned change:

- Analyze the organization and its need for change.
- Create a shared vision and common direction.
- Separate from the past.
- Create a sense of timing (i.e., slow or urgent).
- Support a strong leader role.
- Line up political sponsorship.

- Craft an implementation plan.
- Develop enabling structures.
- Communicate, involve people, and be honest.
- Reinforce and institutionalize the change.

An infinite range of opportunities exists to create change, which depends only on the APN's desires, needs, disposition, and skills. Initiating change requires self-empowerment and leadership. Contributing to productive change creates opportunities to initiate more change through invitations to participate on committees as one develops a reputation for getting things done.

How do APNs manage change in times of turbulence in the health care system?

APNs must possess basic core competencies in advanced practice. Time and practice allow these to be developed more fully. In addition to these competencies, APNs who possess the following attributes will continue to be valuable regardless of changes in the health care system:

- Clinical competence in all facets of advanced nursing practice is required.
- Caring is critical for maintaining stability in an unstable, intimidating system.
- Communication skills are required for successful teamwork.
- Business acumen is needed to understand the costs of health care and help with cost containment.
- Flexibility and creativity are necessary in the changing health care needs, which will continue to evolve.

With emphasis on the access-cost-quality triad, APNs must explore cost-effective opportunities that offer quality health care access to everyone. With the future changes in the health care system, APNs will have the opportunity to have a satisfying practice. In order to survive this turbulence, the following strategies should become a priority of each APN:

- Propose programs that meet gaps in care and save money.
- Make a commitment to action while keeping informed about health care changes.
- Get involved in your practice organization and task redesign efforts.
- Document and report failures of managed care.
- Learn about the economics of your practice.
- Incorporate simple, inexpensive treatments into your practice.
- Identify "designer" practices in your location.
- Develop and evaluate a critical path for a particular patient group.
- Cross-train in areas to benefit patients.
- Lead CQI projects.
- Identify and promote skills.
- Obtain credentials and certification, and display these items on office walls.
- Work with an administrator to evaluate marketing practices.
- Identify your values. Stay informed and make a commitment to action, when necessary.
- Make a decision, take a risk, and pay the price.
- Know the colleagues from other disciplines in your setting.
- Develop supportive interdisciplinary relationships.
- Identify clinicians who offer complementary modalities. Build alliances with them.
- Know your physician colleagues. Educate them and solicit their support on APN issues.

As changes emerge within the health care system, APNs must be receptive to new practice models. We are living in an exciting era of developing globalization. Governmental and corporate policies are dictating the shape of future health models for the APN practice. Our challenge is to develop a new advanced practice for the promotion of health in various geographic populations while improving living conditions. APNs possess the knowledge and skills needed to facilitate such practice models. With more collaborative relationships and productive alliances among health professionals, future challenges can be met.

New Practice Models for APNs: Thinking Outside the Box

2

Mary K. Bailey
Elizabeth Bodie Gross

If you are willing to look at your APN skills and think outside the box, then developing an independent practice might be for you. Health care in the United States serves only a small portion of the people who need care. Over the past 20 years, the growth of medical technologies and treatments has increased exponentially, becoming too complex and expensive for individuals suffering with chronic illnesses to afford or obtain. In order to change health care in the future and improve its quality, we need to think small. Although patients want and need the care of APNs, big business often gets in the way. This chapter offers four new practice APN models that provide exciting ways of dealing with complicated health care cases.

Practice model 1: Geriatric Care Management (GCM) for APNs

In this model, which is the only fully developed model, an APN-GCM contracts with an elderly patient and/or family caregiver to provide care management services for an agreed-upon fee (e.g., an hourly rate or retainer). GCM services are usually for crisis patients in need of advanced health care management or for patients who require management of their long-term care needs so they can remain in their homes, if they are ill or disabled. Patients might be in need of APN-GCM services that allow them to be discharged home safely (following a hospitalization, rehabilitation, or skilled nursing home stay), with their short- and long-term needs appropriately coordinated.

Why Offer GCM Services?

- Most elderly people want to be in their home (as long as possible) even if they require long-term care services. Giving these patients a choice results in better compliance and a more favorable outcome. The majority of the elderly who need GCM services have families who live out of town.

Why Do APNs Make Great Care Managers?

- APNs generally have better access to physicians and other health care providers, and are able to coordinate services for their patients.
- APNs perform comprehensive assessments (and physicals), treat and admit patients to health facilities (when necessary), and order and closely manage medications.
- APNs, as health care experts, assist their patients in navigating acute and long-term care systems more efficiently and easily.

What Services Can APN-GCMs Provide?

Patient care management

After an elderly patient or family caregiver contracts with an APN-GCM, the APN will assess what the patient's health and long-term care needs are, coordinate and manage the services that appropriately meet those needs, provide an ongoing assessment of the client's health care status and needs, and intervene in a crisis when the patient's health condition suddenly changes. The process usually follows these steps:

1. The patient and family caregiver together sign a service contract that stipulates what services will be rendered to the patient.
2. The APN visits the patient and conducts an assessment (usually a focused assessment).
3. A problem list is formulated and prioritized.
4. From the problem list, a care plan is developed and discussed with the elderly patient and his or her family.
5. When necessary, referrals to other licensed personal care and homemaker services are made and coordinated by the APN-GCM

(unless the elderly patient or family member wants to contract these services separately).

6. The APN-GCM acts as a private consultant, available 24 hours a day, 7 days a week, managing all the patient's health and long-term care needs.

7. The APN-GCM maintains communication as long as it is needed with the appropriate providers, including the primary care physician and other health care agencies.

Ongoing care management services

Ongoing care management for frail elderly, disabled, and chronically ill patients who prefer to stay in their own homes, includes the following:

- Weekly, bimonthly, or monthly home visits that assess a patient's health (e.g., diagnosing and treating minor illnesses and medication management) and personal care needs.
- Ongoing assessments and care plan revisions.
- Daily, weekly, or monthly telephone consultations with the elderly and/or family members to address ongoing health care issues.
- With the patient's approval, telephone updates are made with all health and long-term care providers involved in providing care for the elderly patient.
- Advice on where to purchase needed health care products and medications at the lowest cost.

Steps for Developing an APN-GCM Practice

Step 1: The practice plan

- Determine the structure of the practice (e.g., sole proprietorship, S corporation, limited partnership, or other).
- Establish a timeline for the practice.
- Develop marketing strategies.
- Arrange coverage for the APN's vacation or illness ahead of time.
- Outline a plan for securing capital.

Step 2: Marketing

- Develop a brochure that clearly stipulates the type of services being offered, the credentials of the service provider (e.g., your APN résumé), and scenarios for ways in which the service is used by the patient (e.g., the long-term care of a patient trying to cope with a cancer diagnosis).
- Determine the mailing list. For example, the brochure can be mailed with a cover letter to home health and hospice agencies, hospitals, nursing home and rehabilitation center discharge planners, physicians, parish nurses, senior service organizations, community senior services agencies, insurance companies, bank trust departments, and elder law attorneys.

Step 3: Legal issues

- Maintain your APN license.
- Obtain proper care management certifications (e.g., Certified Case Manager [CCM], Certified Managed Care Nurse [CMC], Certified Disability Management Specialist [CDMS], and/or Certified Rehabilitation Nurse [CRC]).
- Review your state's scope of practice for APNs.
- Secure a professional liability insurance policy to cover APN services, care management services, and general business liability.
- Review all contracts and legal forms with legal counsel for proper compliance with practice laws.
- Develop patient files, and include signed contracts, release forms, and accurate, current, and meticulous progress notes.

Step 4: Billing issues

- Establish a billing process using accounting software that provides the capability to maintain proper patient and business financial information.
- Do monthly billing to the elderly patient, family caregiver, third-party payer, trust department, or long-term care insurer.
- Invoice services rendered on behalf of patients, based on the service contract, which include, but are not limited to, telephone

time, travel time, and home visits. For accounting purposes, this should be recorded in 10- or 15-minute increments. Current rates vary nationally, but most nurse case management charges range from between $70 an hour to $125 an hour.

- Become familiar with and follow standard accounting practices.
- Secure the advice of a tax accountant.
- Conduct business audits every 2 to 3 years.

Is Help Available?

Online help for geriatric care managers can be found on the National Association of Professional Geriatric Care Managers' Web site at www.caremanager.org.

Is This a Viable Practice Model for APNs?

Each day nearly 6,000 Americans turn 65 years old. In 10 years, that number will increase to 10,000 Americans each day. As the baby boom becomes the "senior boom," the need for APN-GCMs will explode. Based on patient requirements, an APN-GCM can handle from 5 to 10 patients simultaneously, billing $1,000 to $3,000 per month. Depending on the practice model, it may take a few years to develop a substantial patient base; however, many APN-GCMs subcontract their services to hospitals, physician practices, long-term care providers (e.g., rehabilitation and skilled nursing facilities), home health care agencies, and outpatient clinics to supplement their practices.

Practice model 2: Occupational health APNs

This model is based on occupational health APNs subcontracting their services to small businesses, factories, grain elevators, department store chains, and offices that do not have the adequate resources and/or cannot afford their own occupational health department to meet the needs of their employees.

Why Offer Occupational Health Services?

Today, the primary expense for employers is health care coverage for their employees and retirees. For example, one hospital stay for an employee who suffers a heart attack can cost thousands of dollars to the employer's health care plan and result in the loss of the employee's productivity, require payment for sick time and short-term disability expenses, and necessitate the development of a *back-to-work program* in order for this employee to return to work and be productive. Subcontracting with an on-site occupational health APN is cost effective and convenient, and provides quality primary care service. Ultimately, the employer and employee both win.

What Services Can Occupational Health APNs Provide?

On a scheduled basis, an occupational health APN provides on-site primary care medical management of acute and chronic illnesses, illness prevention and health promotion activities, new employee and annual physicals, disaster and emergency planning, and telephone triage. Referrals are made for drug and alcohol rehabilitation, unemployment case management, and family social work management. The following steps can be used to develop a plan for an occupational health service:

1. Make an initial on-site assessment of the plant/business.
2. Based on assessment findings, generate a problem list with possible interventions.
3. Discuss program and service options with management and employees.
4. Develop a plan of care outlining how services are evaluated on an ongoing basis.

Steps for Developing an Occupational Health APN Practice

Step 1: The practice plan

- The plan outlines how the practice is structured (e.g., sole proprietorship, S corporation, limited partnership, or other). Outline plans for securing capital.

Step 2: Marketing

- A brochure explains the services the occupational health APN provides, the cost benefits of occupational health care, and the

advantages of a positive business culture. The brochure with a cover letter is mailed to members of the local chamber of commerce, potential clients found in the Yellow Pages, and plants/ businesses in the community identified by a windshield survey.
- Telephone calls and visits are made to prospective clients.

Step 3: Legal issues

- Maintain your APN license.
- Review and adhere to your state's scope of practice for APNs.
- Follow your state's requirements for license or certification as an occupational health nurse (if necessary for an APN).
- Follow recommendations for best practices, consultations in occupational health, clinical guidelines, and protocols for practice from the American Association of Occupational Health Nurses (AAOHN).
- Consult a lawyer specializing in worker's compensation and occupational health cases to determine liability and assist in developing a contract.
- Secure a professional liability insurance policy to cover the delivery of APN services, occupational health services, and general business liability.
- Review all contracts and legal forms with legal counsel to ensure proper compliance with state laws.
- Develop patient files, and include signed contracts, release forms, and accurate, current, and meticulous progress notes.

Step 4: Billing issues

- Establish a billing process using accounting software that provides the capability to maintain proper patient and business financial information.
- Do monthly billing to contracted plants and businesses.
- Invoice all services rendered on behalf of the patient, based on the service contract, which includes, but is not limited to, telephone time, travel time, supplies, and home visits. For accounting purposes, these should be recorded in 10- or 15-minute increments.

- Become familiar with and follow standard accounting practices.
- Secure the advice of a tax accountant.
- Conduct business audits every 2 to 3 years.

Is Help Available?

Online help for nurse practitioner occupational health consultation is available from www.aaohn.org. Information about state licensure for occupational health is available at www.ncsbn.org. Information about the requirements for state certification for occupational health is available at www.abohn.org/certif.htm. The National Institute of Occupational Safety and Health (NIOSH) offers training for occupational health professionals at its education and research centers (see www.cdc.gov/niosh/centers.html).

Practice model 3: School health APNs

As the occupational health model suggests, an APN can contract with a school district or private schools (e.g., high schools and community colleges) that do not provide but need part- or full-time health care services for their students.

Why Offer School Health Services?

- Many children in underserved rural and urban public schools, along with children attending private schools, have no available health care (especially primary and/or specialized pediatric care).
- Most schools are financially stressed and choose not to afford full-time school nurses.
- Students miss school because of delinquent school physicals and immunizations.
- Students miss school because of an illness that could have been prevented.
- Students miss participating in athletics when their sports physicals are delinquent.

How Are APNs Beneficial for School Health?

- APNs can diagnose and treat acute and chronic illnesses.
- APNs have proven cost effective in providing primary care services.
- APNs provide quality health care and disease prevention.
- On-site primary health care, provided by the APN, is more convenient, less expensive, and of better quality for parents, students, faculty, and staff.

What Services Can School Health APNs Provide?

School health APNs visit schools on a part- or full-time basis to provide the intermittent management of chronic illnesses, the diagnosis and treatment of acute illnesses, the management of pregnancies, disease prevention, and health promotion. They also administer kindergarten, fifth-grade, and high-school entrance physicals, sports physicals, new faculty and staff physicals, and teacher and staff annual physicals. Additional services include consultation and guidance for faculty regarding student health problems; disaster and emergency planning; health fairs for students, faculty, and staff; teacher and staff health screenings; the development of staff and faculty protocols for medication distribution; and the management of asthma, diabetes, and seizure disorders. The following steps can be used to develop a plan for school health services:

1. Faculty, administration, and families complete a school health assessment survey to identify student, faculty, and staff needs.
2. The APN reviews the survey results and discusses possible interventions with faculty, administration, and family representatives.
3. A plan of services is developed that includes a consideration of how services are evaluated.

Steps for Developing a School Health APN Practice

Step 1: The practice plan

- Develop and structure a practice plan to present to school boards. Outline plans for financial considerations.

Step 2: Marketing

- Develop a brochure that clearly stipulates the type of APN services offered, and the health advantages and cost benefits of service. Enclose a résumé of your past experience, education, and accomplishments.
- Mail the brochure and a cover letter to the superintendent of schools. Develop a power point presentation and present it to the parent/teacher organization and the school board. Outline the advantages, services, and costs of employing a school APN.

Step 3: Legal issues

- Maintain your APN license.
- Review and adhere to your state's scope of practice for APNs.
- Maintain certification as an APN (Family Nurse Practitioner [FNP] or Pediatric Nurse Practitioner [PNP]).
- Follow your state's requirements for a licensed APN school nurse.
- Secure a professional liability insurance policy to cover the delivery of APN services, school health services, and general practice liability.
- Consult a lawyer specializing in child and family law to determine liability and assist in writing a contract.
- Develop patient files, and include signed contracts, release forms, and accurate, current, and meticulous progress notes.

Step 4: Billing issues

- Establish a billing process using accounting software with the capability to maintain proper client and business financial information.
- Bill contracted schools monthly.
- Invoice all services rendered on behalf of the students, faculty, and staff, based on the service contract. An hourly rate is charged, depending on the geographic area, with extra charges for additional services.
- Become familiar with and follow standard accounting practices.
- Secure the advice of a tax accountant.
- Conduct business audits every 2 to 3 years.

Is Help Available?

Online help for school health APNs can be found for each state at www.nasn.org, the Web site of the National Association of School Nurses (NASN), an affiliate organization of the American Nurses Association (ANA). Practice guidelines and protocols are located at www.aap.org, the Web site of the American Academy of Pediatrics (AAP). Information about school nurse certification is available at www.nbcsn.com/national, the Web site of the Board for Certification for School Nurses Inc. (BCSN). Individual state requirements for licensure are found at each state's board of education Web site.

Practice model 4: APN practice for the uninsured/underinsured

This model is based on the APN-GCM model. It is our belief that both the model for managing skilled and personal care for the ill, disabled, and elderly and the model for providing care services are successful in the home. In every community, there are scores of individuals with no health care coverage, yet they are suffering with health needs and concerns; they are scarcely alleviated by the ever growing health care information and advertising offered by the media and Internet. Sadly, this information adds to the confusion and misunderstanding that already exists among the general population about their health. There is a need for sound health education, personal consultation, and low-tech, simple diagnostic procedures and treatments for all healthy individuals, much of which can be done in the home.

Why Offer an APN Practice for the Uninsured/Underinsured?

- The uninsured/underinsured individuals would have access to health care and disease prevention, and receive treatment for minor illnesses in their home.
- The APN can arrange for referrals to providers who treat the more complicated illnesses outside the patient's home.
- The APN's services provide the uninsured and underinsured a lower cost alternative for quality primary care services in their own familiar setting.

What Services Can APNs Provide?

- The APN assesses the patient's health by using a health assessment or risk identification survey, and by performing a focused history and physical examination.
- Screening laboratory tests (such as a urinalysis, a chemistry panel, a lipid panel, or a strap test) are collected and sent to a laboratory.
- Minor illnesses are diagnosed and treated.
- Preemployment physicals are performed.
- Health education is provided based on the health assessment.
- Patients are encouraged to assist in planning their own care.

Steps for Developing an APN Practice for the Uninsured/Underinsured

Step 1: The practice plan

- Develop a plan outlining how the practice is structured (e.g., sole proprietorship, S corporation, limited partnership, or other), how financial resources needed to establish the practice are secured, how laboratory testing services are accessed, and how prescriptive authority in the state of the practice is regulated.

Step 2: Marketing

- Develop a brochure that clearly stipulates the type of services offered, and the health advantages and cost of the service. Provide evidence of the APN's competency (e.g., credentials and résumé).
- Identify patients who access service through personal referral. These might include musicians, pizza deliverers, kitchen workers, underachieving college graduates, farmers, or nonunion laborers. Develop a brochure (e.g., APN résumés) that clearly stipulates the type of service, the cost, and the person offering the service.

Step 3: Legal issues

- Maintain your APN license.
- Review and follow your state's scope of practice for APNs.

- Maintain certification as an APN (FNP and adult health practitioner).
- Secure a professional liability insurance policy to cover the delivery of APN services and general practice liability.
- Have the patient sign permission for performing an invasive procedure, for example, having blood work drawn (e.g., venipuncture).
- Follow all approved practice guidelines and protocols for adult health.
- Consult a lawyer specializing in health care issues to develop contracts, permission-to-treat forms, and release forms.
- Develop patient files, and include signed contracts, release forms, and accurate, current, and meticulous progress notes. All patient information is kept confidential and stored at a secure location.

Step 4: Billing issues

- Invoice services on a fee-for-service basis that is paid at the time of service.
- Prepay all laboratory costs.
- Charge for telephone calls, beginning at a minimum of 10 minutes followed by 15-minute intervals.
- Consult a tax accountant for the proper reporting of practice income.
- Provide receipts to patients for payment of APN services and written reports of assessment findings.
- Obtain accounting software that maintains the proper patient and practice financial information.
- Follow standard accounting practices.
- Conduct business audits every 2 to 3 years.

Is Help Available?

The American Academy of Ambulatory Care Nursing (AAACN) (www.aaacn.org), an organizational affiliate of the ANA, offers certification as an ambulatory care nurse. However, it is necessary to determine if your state's model requires a retainer-based APN collaborative relationship with a physician.

Strategic Planning for Success

3

Trish Goudie

How do APNs lay the groundwork for successful strategic planning?

What is strategic planning? Why is it necessary for a successful nursing practice? How does it work? Who makes it happen? This chapter will answer these questions and assist you in creating a strategic plan for the APN.

Strategic planning is a continuous systematic process of making decisions with the greatest possible knowledge of the current environmental influences, the effects on the future, the determination of efforts necessary to carry out those decisions, and the evaluation of the results of these decisions against the expected outcomes through systematic feedback mechanisms.

Why should APNs do strategic planning? In this era of dynamic economic forces and changing future trends, successful organizations use strategic planning to find ways to secure their place in a competitive environment. APNs, whether they are entrepreneurs establishing their own businesses or those working within organizations, should plan their own future, particularly in response to the many changes in health care.

What is the process of strategic planning?

How does strategic planning start? How often are updates necessary? The following sections provide a guide for the development of a strategic plan for an APN practice. Strategic planning involves an environmental analysis, a strategic plan, and the development of a time frame to complete the process. Strategic planning involves several steps:

1. Planning the process
2. Developing the mission statement
3. Conducting the external assessment
4. Conducting the internal assessment
5. Setting goals and priorities
6. Developing strategies to achieve the goals
7. Developing the implementation plan
8. Evaluating the outcomes

Planning the Process

First, decide who is going to do which tasks in the planning process, the way data will be collected, the time frame for each task, the schedule for meetings, and the timeline for completing the strategic planning process.

Developing the Mission Statement

The mission statement serves as the guide for an APN practice. It includes the philosophy, values, goals, and priorities of the business. If a mission statement for the practice already exists, then review it for accuracy and relevancy. If no mission statement exists, then create one. Answering the following questions can assist you in this process:

- What is the philosophy of the business (values/beliefs)?
- What is the purpose of the practice (reason for existence)?
- What are the objectives? What will be accomplished by the practice? (State specific measurable outcomes.)

Some practices opt to have a philosophy statement as a separate section. The example outlined here provides a separate section in the mission statement for the philosophy, purpose, and objectives.

Mission Statement Example

Philosophy.   We believe that all women are entitled to health care that will result in the best possible outcomes during the provision of maternal/newborn nursing care.

Purpose.   The purpose of the practice is to provide compassionate, evidence-based nursing care to women throughout the perinatal period.

Objectives.   To decrease the incidence of failure to progress in first-stage labor by 10%.

Conducting the External Assessment

This step of the process requires considerable time and effort to effectively research the environmental factors that have an impact on the practice. This step is sometimes referred to as an *environmental scan.* Proposed elements of the external assessment include the following:

- **Economic factors.**   Although it might seem unlikely that a practice in Anytown, USA, would be affected by global trends, it is essential that both a micro- and macroanalysis of economic factors be conducted. The macroanalysis should include both domestic and worldwide economic influences, and their effects on health care providers and consumers, the workforce, and the payers (private, public, and government). The microanalysis should include an examination of state and local government and business climates, unemployment rates, gains/losses of local businesses, and payer coverage of the target population (public, private, and government).
- **Political factors.**   The regulatory environment can change according to the political party in power; therefore, it is essential to be aware that national, state, and local elections can directly affect health care delivery. Some health care issues are highly politicized (e.g., abortion, sex education, contraceptive services, and assisted suicide), which will influence the long-term planning for a health care practice. Be aware of how national and local political factors will affect an APN practice.

- **Market trends.** These should be examined at the national, state, and local level. Some parts of the country have been more readily accepting of alternative care delivery models, which can provide important data for a new practice seeking to address local needs. The following should be included in the analysis:
  - ➤ **Payer marketing.** Promoting services and fee structures to business groups
  - ➤ **Packaged services marketing.** Packaging all services in one center (e.g., a primary care clinic, WIC clinic, or well child clinic)
  - ➤ **Program-focused marketing.** Addressing broader concepts such as women's hospitals and health services and health promotion centers
- **Technology trends.** The joke is that the latest technical toy purchased is obsolete before it leaves the store. Health care technology is constantly changing, and the savvy strategic planner will be up-to-date on the latest advances in biomedical and information systems that affect health care delivery.
- **Social/lifestyle trends.** The changing demographics of American society have had an impact on the delivery of health care in this country. As the baby boomers age, health care options and delivery are altered to fit their needs. What are the current trends? Be sure to examine local as well as national statistics, and how they may affect the APN practice.
- **Regulatory factors.** The following factors are essential:
  - ➤ State agency regulating the APN (most often, it is the state board of nursing)
  - ➤ Statutes/rules relating to nursing practice
  - ➤ State agency regulating prescriptive authority, if applicable
  - ➤ Occupational Safety and Health Administration (OSHA) rules
  - ➤ Environmental Protection Agency (EPA) rules for hazardous waste and water, and air/soil pollution
  - ➤ Food and Drug Administration (FDA) control of diagnostic and treatment procedures and substances
  - ➤ State laws/rules regarding laboratory testing

➤ State laws affecting reimbursement

➤ State agency(ies) regulating health care facilities

• **Competition/institution image.**   Who is the competition? How is the competition similar to the APN practice? How is it different? Is there a niche that the APN practice fills? How are APNs viewed in the health care community? To appraise the competition, research hospital utilization data (such as the number of patient-days and percent of occupancy), and look at the health care provider mix. Your practice image may be assessed by qualitative measures such as patient satisfaction, employee satisfaction, and community satisfaction surveys. The stability of health care provider practices or the retention rates and the Joint Commission on the Accreditation of Healthcare Organizations (JCAHO) are useful quantitative measures (Simms, Price, & Ervin, 2000).

• **Workforce trends.**   This analysis includes information about local, state, and national workforce trends. What is the supply and demand of health care providers? How are providers distributed? Are there unfilled vacancies, or is there oversaturation? What is the status of the *pipeline* for providers, that is, students enrolled in health care provider education programs? Information is available from governmental agencies (e.g., the state board of nursing), professional organizations, and educational institutions (Simms et al., 2000).

Conducting the Internal Assessment

The internal assessment looks at the strengths and limitations of the business. This step should include an examination of the organizational culture, communication, and demographics of the business. For the independent practitioner, include any volunteers (unpaid assistance) and community contacts that work closely with the business.

Setting Goals and Priorities

Goals are determined by matching the strengths and weaknesses of the business with environmental threats and opportunities (Simms et al.,

2000). Goals must be written down, measurable, and specific as to when they will be attained.

Developing Strategies to Achieve the Goals

This step involves the development of the strategies (decisions made to implement the mission statement) needed to achieve the goals and objectives of the plan. Some strategies are easily determined, whereas others require sequential development or radical change. At this point, the aim is to have a list of realistic strategies for each goal. Select the strategies and alternatives that best fit your practice's mission statement and philosophy. The end result will be a realistic plan for the completion of each goal.

Developing the Implementation Plan

This final step is where the tactics (actions to implement the strategy) are determined for each goal and a specific completion date is set. Some goals may be incremental, requiring checkpoints along the timeline to assess progress.

Evaluating the Outcomes

Evaluation is an ongoing process. The plan should be constantly evaluated to assess the effectiveness of the strategies. Additionally, the mission statement (philosophy, purpose, and objectives) should be evaluated annually and revised as needed. A modified external analysis should be conducted according to the needs of the practice (at least yearly), and changes to the plan should be made as a result of relevant findings.

Who can help with the strategic planning process?

This can seem like a daunting process for an independent practitioner, especially for someone with no business experience. However, planning is vital to the success of the venture. Advisors are available in the community to assist in the process, so be sure to consult the following people:

- Attorney
- Accountant
- Retired managers who have great experience and perspective
- Practice management consultant
- Insurance agent
- Physicians
- Hospital leaders
- Community partners

Merging the Professional and Business Models for APN Practices

4

Ann Glasgow

How are the business model and professional model differentiated?

Health care professionals have faced unprecedented challenges over the past few years. The predominant challenge has been in the emerging access-cost-quality triad for those seeking health care and for those delivering the services. The health professional must be concerned with traditional values of service, advocacy, altruism, and autonomy. Many of these come in direct conflict with the emerging triad due to the constantly growing profit-oriented health care system.

The traditional business model is concerned with profits, competition, and the best maneuvers to achieve glowing dollar returns on investments. This produces an inherent clash between business and the traditional role of the health professional. With the emergence of the entrepreneurial spirit among many APNs, elements of the business model are now central to the success of a practice. Successful APN practice models merge the values of both models while resolving the issues of the access-cost-quality triad.

How do these models affect the APN practice?

The APN practice must be based on both models whether it is in an independent or contracted position. Regardless of the practice, the APN is concerned with meeting the demands established by the access-cost-quality triad. A direct result of the business model is the choice to assume responsibilities for the business components of service delivery. Having responsibility for all practice financial liabilities is a key factor. In the contracted position, the APN is a salaried employee who does not carry the financial burdens of the practice.

What should APNs consider before entering an independent practice?

APNs are registered in the states in which they practice and require no business license for entering an independent practice. Because the individual state nurse practice law and regulating bodies dictate the scope of practice for the APN, before opening an independent practice, a meeting with this officiating body is considered a number-one priority to ensure against practice conflicts.

Many APNs going into an independent practice are faced with barriers, which include the following:

- Objection by other professional health care providers in the community due to the threat of losing patients
- Reimbursement denials by insurance companies and managed care plans designed only to reimburse physicians
- Legal protection denied for reimbursements for those procedures also performed by physicians
- Denial of referral arrangements for necessary diagnostic testing, describing the APN as an "unauthorized provider"
- Denial to admit APNs as partners in organized medicine
- Difficulty obtaining hospital privileges
- Not receiving patient payments at the time of visit and the inability to obtain reimbursements from patient insurers

In states where restrictions overwhelm an APN's opportunity to enter an independent practice, many have gone with a collaborating contracted physician. In such instances, the APN should consider developing a careful business plan for his or her own practice contract. If the APN has a limited business background to make a plan, selected key consultants should be engaged so as to ensure success.

What factors should APNs include when considering a business plan for an independent practice?

In preparation for a successful independent practice, APNs should ask the following questions:

- What is the target population? How will these patients be reached? What services need to be offered for the practice to flourish? What type of marketing is necessary to reach the target goals?
- What type of organization is the best? Who will run the organization? What type of management expertise is required?
- Where are start-up funds found? How are revenues generated? What are the projected revenues and expenses for 1, 3, and 5 years? What is the timeline for the business to be debt free and self-supporting?
- How are reimbursements with insurance and managed care companies established? What is required to submit the appropriate forms to receive reimbursements expediently?
- What staff is required to operate the practice? What scope of services is offered? What type of equipment is needed? What federal and state regulations must be observed? What are the fees for these applications?
- Where can financing for the initial expenditures be acquired? Will the loan institution require a financial statement and projected business plan?
- What must be done to incorporate the practice? Does the practice aim to have 501c(3) status from the Internal Revenue Service (IRS)? Does a corporation or partnership need to be formed? What type of corporation is needed to contract with a collaborating physician? Does that differ from structuring a corporation with a physician as a participant? Can a corporation be formed with a physician as a professional corporation or does a limited liability corporation fit the practice better?
- Will the practice have advisors or a board of directors?
- Who will make up the practice's board of directors? Who are the most likely members for the board in the community? Should there be community involvement on the board?

- What is required from the IRS and state tax commission? Is the practice a nonprofit, tax-exempt organization? What is the purpose (business activities, funding sources, board composition, and services) of the corporation?

What is the difference between an employee and independent contractor?

Is the APN an employee or independent contractor in the practice? As an independent contractor, a physician contracts with the APN and bills services "incident to" the physician services, which means the physician is directly in a supervisory position. The APN may obtain a provider number independent of the physician, which allows billing to occur under that number for services directly performed.

APNs have established successful practices with contracted collaborative physicians. If risk is not a factor, there is no limit to what an APN can accomplish:

- An APN, working as an independent contractor,
  - ➤ Makes a profit or suffers loss.
  - ➤ Is hired to complete a certain job and is liable for incompletion damages.
  - ➤ Works for a number of firms or physicians at the same time.
  - ➤ Publicly advertises the APN services that are available.
  - ➤ Pays for expenses including the equipment and location.

- The following are factors that demonstrate an employer-employee relationship:
  - ➤ The employer is in control.
  - ➤ The APN may be terminated.
  - ➤ The employer furnishes the equipment and staff.
  - ➤ The APN must perform work required by the employer.
  - ➤ Training is received from the employer and the APN is required to follow instructions.
  - ➤ The employer establishes work time and the type of position, either full-time or part-time.
  - ➤ The employer pays business expenses.

➤ The APN employee's income, paid by salary or the hour, week, or month, may be determined by clock-in procedures along with other staff. Negotiate. (Do all the professional staff members clock in?)

➤ The APN does not hire, supervise, or pay assistants or licensed practical (vocational) nurses who assist daily with medical procedures.

Who cares about the type of APN practice?

The main concern of the state regulation body for the APN is whether or not the APN is practicing within the scope of practice dictated by law. Many APNs face administrative reprimands, suspensions, and probation due to violations of regulations mandated in state statutes and regulating bodies. Know the state statutes and regulations prior to opening a practice and observe them. Good documentation of your experiences is important.

Business owners and tax regulating agencies (federal and state) are concerned with the type of relationship within the practice. These agencies want a clear description of the relationship to ensure that the appropriate taxes are paid. In the employer-employee role, the employer has the responsibility to withhold and pay payroll taxes, Social Security, Medicare contributions, premiums for unemployment, and worker's compensation insurance. In an independent contractor role, each party is responsible for paying taxes and insurance premiums. The practice owner wants a clear description of the relationship to avoid negative sanctions imposed by taxing agencies.

Practice owners are concerned about the relationship with the APN. They may want control of the work performed. On the other hand, they may believe the APN will inspire commitment and loyalty. The owner may also prefer the increased flexibility that short-term APNs offer rather than hiring full-time employees. Establish a clearly defined relationship.

As an APN, you need to consider which avenue to take. Do you enjoy the tax deductions available to an independent contractor and the freedom to contract with several different practices? Consider employee status if you dislike the hassle of filing tax forms, paying taxes, and keeping track of withholdings on a quarterly basis.

What facts should APNs consider when contracting to a practice?

According to the American Academy of Nurse Practitioners (AANP), the following tips should be carefully considered prior to contracting to a practice:

- Determine if the position is salaried or based on a per-hour, per-day, or per-patient contract.
- Based on production figures, it is possible to obtain some estimate of your net worth to the practice. If your income expectation is higher than the costs incurred, the practice probably cannot afford you.
  - ➤ The APN who is expected to take call must determine what percent of other provider salaries in the practice are attributed to this activity. The APN expects to receive a similar percentage if taking call is rotated with other providers.
  - ➤ If the APN is expected to conduct hospital rounds, revenues to the practice are figured into the APN's salary/payment estimates.

Benefits to Consider

- If the APN is salaried, negotiated benefits (in addition to salary) include
  - ➤ Health insurance.
  - ➤ Vacation (at least 3 to 4 weeks per year).
  - ➤ Sick leave (generally 2 weeks or 1 day per month per year).
  - ➤ Travel allowance if the APN is expected to make house calls.
  - ➤ Continuing education allowance and leave. Going to one to two conferences per year is not inappropriate. Include in this

allowance airfare, room, and food for at least one national conference. An allowance of $1,500 to $2,500 for this purpose is reasonable.
> Malpractice insurance.
> Professional organization memberships.
> Office subscriptions to the appropriate nurse practitioner journals.

Practice Expectations to Consider

- Determine if you will be able to practice to the full extent of your scope of practice.
- Check for barriers more stringent than those existing in state law or regulation.
- Determine that you will not be expected to practice beyond the scope of your practice.

Other Cautions

- Do not bite off more than you can chew.
- A new nurse practitioner needs mentoring and more time per patient than an experienced APN. Take this into account when negotiating your first contract.

An attorney should draw up the legal contract used by an independent contractor so that all aspects of the practice are included (e.g., those listed in the previous tips). Be sure agreements between the two parties are clearly written and mutually understood so no future misunderstandings that might lead to adverse action will arise.

What avenues can APNs take to increase practice profits?

In the area of profit, business components are deeply involved with the health professional model. For the practice to become successful, profit generation must be one of the highest priorities. An APN who uses time efficiently is valuable in generating income in a medical practice. A working knowledge of business practice is essential—for example, receiving maximum reimbursement, keeping abreast of billing rules established and changed for coding, and diligently taking initiative for reaching the business budget.

To achieve maximum revenues within a practice, APNs can do the following:

- Increase the number of patient visits per workday.
- Increase the average charge for a patient visit by better coding and accurate recording of billable services.
- Charge for all services provided. Include adequate, accurate documentation for necessary procedures and treatments.
- Increase attentiveness to items that are not payable by insurers.
- Increase legislative involvement to attain reimbursement for APN services at the same fee schedule physicians enjoy.
- Reward each provider who performs well with an incentive based on gross charges.

To achieve the previous goals, acquire business-medical computer software that interrelates all aspects. Many systems are available that document medical information and business data required for accurate patient billing. The Logician system, just one of many software programs, does a wonderful job documenting and coding, and provides better service billing to include current and accurate codes (at the fingertips of the provider) with matching diagnoses. It contains a pharmaceutical program that provides the accurate prescription of medications with a cross-reference to other current medications used by the patient in a printed form, thus decreasing pharmacy errors.

On the business side, to review revenues and expenses, the practice accounting program can be accessed as often as the provider deems necessary. Inefficient areas of service are quickly identified and dealt with so that changes prevent the loss of revenue. A daily business log is an invaluable tool for accessing the status of revenues and providing accountability for staff members responsible for charges and deposits. Monthly logs give an overall look at monthly expenses. These logs are separated by departments and the services offered, so corrections are easily made. As a result, expenses and revenues are broken out to determine if certain services should be continued or if the operation cost for the department includes too many charges and deposits.

How do APNs measure success?

APNs, from a professional model viewpoint, define success by delivering quality health care and seeing satisfied patients. Increasing revenues, decreasing expenditures, and increasing productivity with cost management and profitability define the business model viewpoint.

Merging the business model with the health professional model is difficult, but with the changes in the health care system, regardless of the provider, it has become inevitable and necessary for the survival of a practice. Providers have little choice but to merge their practices into a business model that provides better access, lower costs, and higher quality for all patients. APNs are the best resource for adapting practices into this model. All health providers must collaborate in erasing barriers that affect this model.

The professional and business models of health care delivery are currently able to merge into a successful health care system that has the following key attributes:

- A clearly defined philosophy of how the practice views success (focusing on vision and accomplishment).
- Agreement among those involved in the management of practice philosophy and goals.
- A plan to achieve success as defined by the group. If you fail to plan, you plan to fail.
- Clearly defined, measurable short- and long-term goals.
- A continuous collection and review of data to monitor the practice performance—for example, provider revenue and expense per practice department, patient volume, the type of patients, referrals, clinical outcomes, patient satisfaction, the breakdown of insurers seen by a practice, reimbursement patterns, coding profiles, and the average time of claims and collection rates every 30, 60, and 90 days.

- Quality patient care and patient satisfaction continuously monitored and embraced by the practice.
- Good leadership, practicing sound medical and administrative decisions (such as a respected physician associated in collaborative association with an equally respected APN).
- Involvement in all aspects of running the practice.
- Clear lines of communication and trust among providers of a group practice relayed to all members, and a focus on professional ability and productivity.
- Knowledge of the practice market. Devise a plan that includes the demographics of the community, the structure and politics of the physician-APN community, and the range of services offered to patients and the practice.
- A commitment to hiring and retaining the best physicians, APNs, nurses, medical assistants, administrators, and support staff.
- An investment in realistic equipment and technology is imperative to maintaining a balance between income and expenses.

Success is measured by the yearly continuation of a quality practice. Successful practices are sustainable when committed leadership plans carefully with a clear vision. When this vision is shared, the practice is empowered by the commitment of everyone involved.

Credentialing and Continuing Education

5

Ann Glasgow

What is the purpose of having rules and regulations for APNs?

Public health, safety, and welfare rules and regulations exist to protect citizens. They set the minimal requirements for APNs to practice competently and safely. The primary methods of regulation include credentialing and continuing education. Following their education in an accredited master's degree program for Advanced Practice Nursing, APNs should be able to meet the requirements for national and state credentialing at the level they want to practice. Credentialing occurs at two different levels: licensure and certification.

How does an APN obtain licensure?

Licensure is a legal process that takes place at the state level in accordance with the Nurse Practice Act in the state where the APN wants to practice. The board responsible for licensure (which in most states is the state board of nursing) establishes clearly defined qualifications, the scope of practice, prescriptive authority, and the use of the APN title. Laws for licensure vary greatly from state to state.

Currently, the predominant trend is for a nurse with a bachelor's degree to graduate from an accredited Master of Science nursing educational program and acquire national certification. Prior to graduation, the APN needs to contact the state board of nursing or official licensing board to apply and obtain requirements specific to that state. The process takes time. Plan ahead; eliminate barriers that postpone your ability to practice. A temporary permit can carry you in many states until a license is obtained. Contact the licensing agency for the specific state in which you want to practice. (See Appendix 2 for a list by state.)

Many licensing agencies require periodic renewals accompanied by the documentation of continuing education and clinical experience. Find out what is expected by the state in which you are practicing and keep a verifiable record of renewal data. Compile a filing system that includes documents describing the types of programs you attended, specifying the dates and number of hours.

How does an APN obtain certification?

Certification is the process through which a nongovernmental agency certifies that an APN has met the minimal requirements of professional practice standards. Certification protects the public by ensuring that an APN has achieved basic competency knowledge and skills for a particular area of practice. Apply to the certifying agency for the specific area of practice before graduating from an APN program. Most nongovernmental agencies require that an APN candidate

- Hold an active registered nurse license in the United States or its territories.
- Hold a master's degree or higher in nursing.
- Be prepared in the practice specialty area for which the APN has applied for certification through a master's program or a formal postgraduate master's program in nursing.
- Have graduated from a program offered by a school of nursing granting graduate-level academic credit for all course work.
- Have graduated from a program that includes both didactic and clinical components.
- Have graduated from a program that includes a minimum of 500 hours of supervised clinical practice in the specialty area and role.

Upon graduation, a transcript from the APN's school with the date of graduation and degree obtained will be needed. Once the application process is completed, it takes several weeks to establish a testing date. Some of the agencies have testing dates only twice a year. Be aware of the certifying center deadlines. The American Nurses Credentialing Center (ANCC) test is computerized and has established testing dates at local testing centers. Each agency will send you a copy of testing categories or you can find them on their Web sites. (See Appendix 1 for a list of certifying boards in specific practice areas.)

ANCC certification is valid for 5 years with an option to renew by submitting evidence of continuing education obtained during the 5-year period or by retaking the examination. APNs certified by the American Academy of Nurse Practitioners (AANP) Certification Program may become recertified every 5 years by taking the appropriate examination or by meeting the clinical practice and continuing the recertification education requirements. These requirements include at least 1,000 hours of clinical practice in the area of specialization and 75 contact hours of continuing education relevant to the area of specialization. Other agencies have independent requirements that can be found by contacting their offices. The recertification and credentialing process recognizes initial and sustained competency, and demonstrates the APN's commitment to quality care.

How does an APN prepare for the certification examination?

Many schools offer their graduates review sessions comprised of material and testing similar to the certification exams. The best approach is not to wait until the last moment and try to cram. Start the review process early during the educational phase. Testing manuals and tapes that assist in the review process are available at university bookstores and online at certification sites (e.g., ANCC and AANP). Get them well ahead of time and plan a structured daily study program before taking the exam. If you feel you are not prepared for the exam, cancel the testing date and, for a small fee, reschedule when you have the adequate confidence and knowledge. Several agencies offer review courses that for the most part are beneficial in preparation for these tests. Each group offers tests similar to the exam that is taken on the computer or with pencil. Review groups offering helpful programs include Fitzgerald Health Education Associates and Mary Kellermann Educational Entities. Both can be found on the Internet at the ANCC and AANP sites for certification review materials.

What is the scope of practice for an APN?

The Nurse Practice Act legislated in each state that licenses an APN delineates the standards of practice according to the practice specialty. The general scope of practice, relative to all practices, is the assessment of health status, diagnosis, and case management. An expansion of the scope of practice is obtained with additional training and experience if it falls within the individual state's Nurse Practice Act. To find out the specific standards for your own practice, contact the licensing board. The Nurse Practice Act for each individual state is accessible at each state's Web site. Barriers to the scope of practice for the APN include the lack of third-party reimbursement, prescriptive authority, and hospital admission privileges. Investigate these areas before entering a practice so that the appropriate actions can be taken to ensure that you are practicing within the legal parameters established by your state's licensing body.

What is the importance of continuing education?

Continuing education is a requirement that keeps your professional knowledge current while ensuring the renewal of licensure and recertification in your practice specialty. Continuing formal or self-education is essential for APNs to maintain and expand their level of competency to anticipate their role in health care and delivery, and to expand the body of professional knowledge.

Starting in 2003, 50% of the continuing education requirement for recertification by the ANCC must be from either an ANCC-accredited or-approved provider, or one of the following providers:

- American Academy of Family Practitioners (AAFP)
- AANP
- American Academy of Physicians Assistants (AAPA)
- American College of Nurse Midwives (ACNM)
- Accreditation Council on Continuing Medical Education (ACCME) Category I
- American Psychiatric Nurses Association (APNA)
- National Association of Nurse Practitioners in Women's Health (NPWH)

- National Association of Pediatric Nurse Associates and Practitioners (NAPNAP)

In addition, offerings are accepted as part of the 50% requirement provided by organizations accredited by the ACCME Category I, such as the American Academy of Pediatrics. A majority (51%) of the contact hours/continuing education must be related to your specialty. Other types of continuing education contact hours are accepted for the remaining 49%. An example of the requirements of individual certifying agencies can be found at their Web sites or in the material received at the time of certification. Licensure is also based on specific continuing education requirements that are obtained from your state's licensing board.

Distance learning has become a direct access for APNs who have difficulty finding time to leave their practice. Internet access offers interactive participation in classrooms and educational materials. Suggestions can be found under certifying agencies as part of their services or under their associated links to Web sites for additional educational programs.

Some schools offer opportunities to certified APNs to become certified in other specialty areas or to continue in an APN doctoral program in nursing. More APNs with PhDs are providing direct patient care and assuming roles as academic clinicians. By offering cost-effective teaching methods using interactive technology directed to homes and workplaces, distant learning programs empower the APN with the opportunity to earn advanced professional knowledge. In addition, these programs, which are available at various schools of nursing (e.g., Case Western Reserve University), enable the APN to attend intensive classes several times a year to accomplish an education at the doctoral level. The Internet is a great resource for accessing university admission requirements, registration, and degree criteria.

Financing the Practice   6

Jeani Thomas

What degree of expertise is required for an APN to financially manage a practice?

One of the greatest inherent hazards faced by an APN in a new business is the uncertainty of the business climate. Many hazards are overcome with good financial planning and a realistic look at opportunities. The degree of expertise required by an APN is directly related to his or her previous management experience. The APN may feel comfortable about budgeting, but be uncertain about payroll taxes, retirement, or how to incorporate. To ensure the success of the practice, the business should be developed to include skills that complement the APN's experience.

What financial expertise is expected of an APN?

Although an APN is not expected to be a lawyer or accountant, a reasonable understanding of laws affecting the practice is necessary. Regulations that affect the practice clinically include the Occupational Safety and Health Administration (OSHA) for the handling of hazardous material and the Clinical Laboratory Improvement Amendment (CLIA) for the maintenance of laboratories. Some of the regulations affecting the practice managerially include corporation status, tax law, social security law, payroll taxes, and local ordinances about signage.

The managers of a practice should first hire a trusted accounting firm. Interview several firms. To establish a checklist of what you expect from a firm, look for previous health care accounting, an understanding of contractual allowances, efficiency in reports, and a good understanding of tax law.

An accountant is valuable in advising you regarding attorneys, banks, and bankers who relate best to small service businesses. The accountant may also be aware of insurance carriers in your area who provide fire, accident liability, and other insurance on equipment and property. The accountant sees many numbers and can clue you in on who can advise and offer the best prices for services.

The accounting firm you choose will assist you in starting the tax year for the practice, choosing an accounting method, and setting up journal files. Look for a firm that will assume payroll and will help with the forms employees need to complete when hiring, gathering information (for tax purposes), and paying payroll taxes. In most accounting firms, this service is included for a reduced fee, which is normally less than what the practice could provide for itself.

What must be included in setting up a budget?

Planning is essential in developing an independent practice. Start-up costs range from several hundred to several thousand dollars. Deciding the clientele you plan to serve clarifies the equipment requirements and projected cash flow. A practice that makes home and nursing home visits to Medicare/Medicaid patients might require more money for transportation but less for office equipment. A practice that concentrates on occupational medicine might have extended hours, and need to purchase a spirometry unit and breath alcohol analyzer. A practice that plans to operate as a rural health center will need to meet special guidelines and requirements to perform specific lab tests in the office, such as hemoglobin/hematocrit, and pay for additional equipment, including a microscope. After carefully planning and reviewing the clientele to be served and the essential items required to operate the practice, you are ready to develop a budget. The practice should plan to expand the services provided during the second and third year of operation.

Planning for the financial operation of the practice is projected monthly for the first year and quarterly for the second and third year. The budget helps determine the cost of the services provided, including rent, personnel, supplies, utilities, and indirect expenses, such as depreciation. As the number of patients increases, variable costs increase. Fixed costs, such as rent, utilities, and equipment, remain the same. The patient census grows and the cash flow increases as costs become stable.

Fixed cost charges for services are set at the start-up and then adjusted yearly. Patient service charges are the base for the income.

An accounting firm will assist the practice in determining the numbers to watch daily, weekly, monthly, quarterly, and yearly. The same accounting firm will review and advise the practice on any budget item before including it in the business plan. A responsible accountant can address budget negatives that are overlooked by the practice manager. A good accountant will question figures that look unreasonable and assist in finding answers to the tough questions bankers and funding sources have a habit of asking.

What items are included in the start-up costs?

The start-up costs for an independent practice are reviewed in the following sample business plan.

- Attorney fees
- Incorporation fees
- Accounting firm fees
- Licensure fees
- CLIA lab fees
- Rent plus a deposit for the building
- Deposit to set up phone service and other utilities
- Telephone equipment and installation, pagers, and answering service
- Printing costs, including checks, signage, business cards, and brochures
- Advertising costs—newspaper, radio ads, billboards, open house, and so on
- Reference books and patient educational information
- Equipment for exam rooms, depending on the clientele—exam table, lighting, scales, digital thermometers, sphygmomanometer, measuring tapes, clock, sink, counter, chair, and stool

(continued)

(continued)

- Supplies for exam rooms—table paper, speculums, urine cups, tissues, and Pap kits
- Equipment for the business office—fax, computer, copier, printer, and calculator
- Supplies for the business office—paper, pens, calendars, postage, files, and forms for patient charts and billing
- Equipment for the lab—a microscope, hemoglobin/hematocrit analyzer, breath alcohol analyzer, spirometry unit, and glucometer
- Supplies for the lab—hemocult cards and reagent, rapid pregnancy tests, rapid strep tests, urine dipsticks, and supplies for the lab equipment
- Postage machine
- Interest on borrowed money
- Waiting room furniture
- Petty cash and a contingency fund to operate in an emergency

---

How does the APN obtain funding sources?

Funding comes from federal sources and foundations. Hawkins and Thibodeau (1996) list available funding and grant information:

- Federal funding source information
  - ➤ Commerce Business Daily
  - ➤ Federal Register
  - ➤ Catalog of Federal Domestic Assistance
  - ➤ Annual Register of Grant Support
  - ➤ Federal Grants and Contracts Weekly
  - ➤ Health Grants and Contracts Weekly
- Foundation funding sources
  - ➤ Foundation Directory and Foundation Grants Index
  - ➤ Annual Register of Grant Supports

➤ Foundation News
➤ State directories of foundations
➤ Academic Research Information System Funding Messenger
➤ The Foundation Grants Index
➤ Source Book Profiles
➤ The Catholic Guide to Foundations
➤ Directory of Biomedical and Health Care Grants (serial)

Receiving funding from grants and foundations is time consuming; so are loans from lending institutions and relatives. Frequently, foundations require different forms and information. Once incorporated, the practice may apply for a business loan for start-up and operation costs. The amount of money needed is determined by the budget and includes start-up money and operating funds for a minimum of 3 months. Each member of the practice corporation is required to develop a financial statement and be willing to guarantee the obligations of the corporation in order to borrow money. Most banks will not loan money to new corporations without a personal guarantee and signatures from stockholders, spouses, and relatives (who are actually guaranteeing the loan).

Another financing option is to partner with a corporation to obtain funding, collaboration, and support. The local hospital may partner with the practice. The hospital will benefit by having patients with possible referrals and lab work served in their area. The practice benefits doubly by having financial support and support from the hospital in the community. An APN practice may also partner with a larger practice that shares identical goals. The larger practice might at the moment prefer to remain at another location, but still happily provide part of the equipment, assist with financing, and collaborate with patients. Each of these partners could make the loan interest bearing, defer principle payments, or provide part of the equipment.

What steps are required for setting up third-party reimbursement?

In the beginning, the APN practice may want to partner with a billing service. Like the accounting firm, billing services have many contacts that make it easier to obtain third-party reimbursement. Talk with and interview several billing services before making a decision. Do not decide based on the lowest price. You should look for the following options. Is there electronic billing of all claims? What reports will the practice receive? Will they post payments and make deposits to the bank account? Will the practice receive aging reports from the monthly accounts? Can they determine which payers are slow to pay?

Billing services usually have contacts with various payers and know the payers in your area, know approximately what they pay, and know whom to contact to become a provider. They have contacts with payers on a first-name basis and can call when the provider application is slow to be returned or when a bill is rejected.

The billing service will identify the accounts receivable numbers you should watch on a monthly basis. They also provide productivity reports for each provider based on the amount billed, the number of visits per day or month, and the amount received on the accounts. They understand and can review charts for correct coding, preventing fraud or lost charges. A good billing service is an invaluable tool for your practice.

How does an APN set up a fee schedule?

The practice lists all services to be provided. Before setting fees, carefully study the Current Procedural Terminology (CPT) published and updated yearly by the American Medical Association.

Reviewing the current fee schedules from other area practices provides welcomed business smarts in setting charges. Charges should be updated with new codes and upgraded charges should appear in the annual review. Charges for the practice are adjusted by third-party payers based on the usual and customary charges for the same service in the same area. Medicare has set allowable charges for the services provided. For example, Medicare is billed a charge of $70 for a #99213, an established patient visit. The Medicare allowable charge for a #99213 is $50. Medicare will reimburse the practice at the rate of 80% of the allowable, or $40. The remaining 20% of the allowable, or $10, will be charged to the patient or a secondary insurance. The difference between the charged amount and the allowed amount is referred to as a *contractual allowance.* Therefore, the contractual allowance for this service is $20. When budgeting for the practice, it is very important to understand this method of payment.

Medicaid has set fees that are paid for specific codes. Other forms of insurance, Health Maintenance Organizations (HMOs), and managed care organizations contract with the practice for reduced fee schedules. The prices contracted are normally a discounted amount of the fee schedule, typically 10% to 20%. Some insurers may have set fees for the area. In order to participate in the plan, the practice will need to contract and accept those fees. Practice managers determine the fee schedule.

How is the collection ratio estimated?

The amount collected for services provided by the practice is determined by the allowable amount for the service by the payers. A list of allowable charges for specific billable codes can be obtained from Medicare and Medicaid. Closely monitoring payments from HMOs and other managed care organizations is a requisite.

Monitoring the amount received for a specific code throughout the year alerts the practice to a need for change in the fee schedule. An example of this is a nursing home visit, a #99333. The fee charged for this in the practice is $100. The allowable charge from Medicare is $90. The practice is receiving the maximum allowable from Medicare. As the payments come in from the HMOs and Preferred Provider Organizations (PPOs), the bookkeeper notes that $100 is consistently paid for the visit. At the yearly review of fee schedules, the practice wants to increase the charge 10% to $110. Medicare continues to allow $90, but the insurance carriers might pay up to $110 for the visit.

Charges should not be adjusted down in an attempt to gain market share. Charges for occupational work that is not covered by third-party payers should be negotiated. Occupational work includes physicals, respirator fit tests, and injury care. Employers pay for occupational services in a timely manner with simplified billing techniques. The practice can gain cash flow while building the business, if it is able to provide these types of service. Worker's compensation insurers pay for injury care and follow-up visits.

What should an APN consider to effectively schedule patient visits?

The decision of scheduling patient visits is made by both the provider and practice manager. When a provider is doing extensive chronic illness care, with multiple diagnoses and medications, more appointment time is needed. Walk-in patients with single problems requiring immediate attention are normally scheduled at the rate of three per hour. Complete physicals require a minimum of 30 minutes. Most schedules are a combination of these categories. The provider may note on a patient's follow-up schedule if the next visit should be 15, 20, or 30 minutes. This tells the person scheduling the appointment the prescribed time necessary for the visit.

Sending appointment reminders to the patient improves patient flow and helps the practice establish a patient base. It is helpful to schedule two to three 15-minute slots each day for patients who are sick and need to be seen that day. Many practices schedule patients for same-day visits by scheduling 10 visits for an 8-hour day. Patients are encouraged to call in the morning if they need an unscheduled appointment. They are given a time to come in, which fills the available openings of the scheduled day. Some practices have one provider who schedules walk-ins every morning. The provider is rotated, so the same provider is not always seeing walk-ins.

A combination of the previous methods is the best approach. Providers and managers soon know the practice and the capability of their providers. Additional factors to consider when scheduling include the number of exam rooms available to each provider, the number of personnel in the registration area, and the number of nurses available for patient care. Scheduling expertise can be taught by experienced providers and office managers.

Developing a Marketing Strategy 7

Ann Glasgow

Why market an APN practice?

The marketing for an APN practice is designed to increase patient awareness and use of the services that are offered by the practice. As a professional, an APN has a wealth of information others find helpful and necessary in seeking a better quality of life. Many APNs have built successful practices by promoting their professional image through effective marketing plans. Marketing includes public relations such as advertising, creating brochures, networking, attending meetings of professional groups, giving public talks, and holding private seminars.

What is involved in marketing a practice?

The primary objective of marketing a practice is to share the services and knowledge you have with patients within your community. They are interested in how they can benefit by selecting you as their provider. You should include several points when marketing your practice:

- What services or products are offered by your practice?
- How do the services you offer meet the needs of patients?
- In what way do the services you offer affect how patients feel about themselves and the care they receive? Does your staff show respect to patients? Do you listen to what patients have to say?
- How do the services you offer patients affect future accessibility? Do they feel secure with you as their provider? Do they feel supported by your services? Can they access someone in the practice at all times?

- How convenient are the services you offer? Are they easily attainable? Do patients have a short waiting period? Do you offer personal conveniences within the facility if the waiting room delay is too long?
- Is there a cost advantage in selecting you as their health care provider?
- How will your services affect their overall financial situation? Do they have to pay up front for a visit? Do you accept their insurance? Are you a provider listed on their primary care provider's list?

How do APNs market a practice?

Once you establish your vision for the practice, you need to find good avenues within your community to get the message out to potential patients. The best method for achieving optimal marketing vehicles depends on your marketing budget, target market, services, competition, and message. Since every marketing vehicle costs money, carefully plan your budget for this expense. Assess your target market to reach the highest numbers within the community in need of your services.

Become knowledgeable in the specific services you intend to offer your community so that patients will seek you as their health care provider. In your effort to become established as a primary caregiver in the health care field, you should first achieve the credentials essential to becoming expert in the areas you have chosen. Survey the potential competition within your area and analyze the services they offer, so you can concentrate on services that demonstrate your expertise. Then you are ready to promote and advertise your professional services.

What are the keys to promoting and advertising APN services?

As a professional, you have a wealth of knowledge that others can find helpful. This knowledge is central in the promotion of your patient services:

- Develop a spoken presentation appropriate for any audience. Follow one of these formulas:
  - ➤ Plead the cause. Create dissatisfaction, recommend a remedy, answer the objections that are in the minds of listeners, and ask for action.
  - ➤ Inform. Explain what it is that you will discuss. Tell the audience about the subject, repeat what you told them, and use a conclusion that listeners will remember.
  - ➤ Present a program, a breakthrough, or a piece of new equipment. What is it? What does it do? How do you use it? Why should the listener use it?
  - ➤ Present material. What happened in the past? What is currently happening today? What is expected to happen in the future? What can the listener do about the present and future changes?
- Develop successful news releases for the promotion of your professionalism. Follow these tips:
  - ➤ Keep the copy simple and important looking. Clear copy with good subtitles makes the news release easy to read and interesting.
  - ➤ Use present tense and active verbs. News is sharper and more action oriented in present tense.
  - ➤ Write from the reader's viewpoint. Make the story important to readers. Take the news release and relate it to their interests.
  - ➤ Bring technical features to life with colorful adjectives. Whenever possible, use words that convey pictures.
  - ➤ Number the features/benefits. For example, if you are writing about a new health breakthrough, list the features/benefits for the reader numerically from 1 to 10.
  - ➤ Use short sentences. For the news release, the maximum sentence length should be 14 to 17 words.
  - ➤ Add personal pronouns whenever possible.
  - ➤ Create an interesting news release that enhances your professional image.

It is possible to increase your professional image with various activities. Use the following suggestions:

- Write a weekly or monthly column for a local newspaper. Include your photo and business address.
- Arrange for appearances on your television station's program about business trends, if possible.
- Offer your professional services as an expert in your professional specialty to the local radio station. Consider the interview or listener call-in formats. Contact your local educational radio stations for this type of publicity.
- Prepare interesting news releases about the latest developments in your professional field. Identify your practice with new developments.
- Serve on worthwhile charities and other well-recognized social activities. Promote your practice as a focal point.
- Prepare slides and films to be shown at local schools. Present the material in person or ask a personable staff member to make the presentation. Be personally identified with the material. Check with the pharmaceutical company representatives who visit your practice for available slides and videos covering the key topics you want to present.

Marketing is the key to promoting your professional practice. The following secrets are important steps in successful marketing:

- The credentials you acquire during school and certifications prior to practicing lay the foundation for the services you offer as an APN.
- It is critical to believe in yourself as a professional APN.
- A total commitment to your vision with established reachable goals is important for achieving success.
- Understanding the principles of business is a must. Continue your education with materials that improve your skills.
- Using your vision guidelines, establish daily goals that are easily attainable. Daily focus is helpful in reaching long-term goals. Be

sure to keep a current journal in which you write down your goals. Reviewing them helps plan the future.
- Your vision lists the goals that define your overall plan. Review and critique your achievement.
- To achieve your goals, establish a schedule and adhere to it. Persist and you will reach your vision.
- Persistence is the key to reaching your vision. Do not let someone steal your dream. Failure is just one more step to success.

How do APNs build referrals to their practice?

Networking is a vital component of every successful marketing plan. Professional colleagues are a major source of referrals. Professionals within your practice area can provide immediate referrals to the services you offer as a specialty. For example, if you have lipid training, any patients with hyperlipidemia problems can be referred to you for management.

Participation in a professional organization provides an audience of professionals who can learn to respect you and serve as a referral source. Getting involved in your community is a characteristic of a good citizen. As an APN, you will educate the community! Performing school physicals and nominal-cost physicals at community centers is a constant referral source.

The managed care environment of a community offers a referral basis that can be tapped by showing the company how you meet their clinical and service expectations. Consider why your practice does not do enough business with a particular company and then market to that group in order to increase your referrals. Offer services such as plant tours that assist in detecting occupational hazards, or look at job requirements and suggest methods that might avoid increased worker's compensation claims. These services have proved invaluable to the managed care group while proving beneficial to the practice. Be creative and knowledgeable about the group among which you are soliciting patients. Whatever method of networking you use, do exceptional work and those involved will remember you.

How do APNs achieve an effective marketing plan for their practice?

Marketing is a continual process of gathering internal and external data to improve your practice and, at the same time, provide information to the target audience about the services being offered. Some practices that have enough income hire a firm to do full-scale marketing and advertising promotion. For those that have limited funds, the staff can collect data. Develop an effective marketing plan using the following:

- Decide on your vision covering the next 3 to 5 years and establish reachable short- and long-term goals.
- Develop a marketing plan to accomplish your goals. Gather and analyze current practice data. (See Appendix 3 for a suggested patient survey of a practice.)
- Gather internal data from the computer information system, concentrating on patient demographics, the number of patients seen over the last 3 years, and patient mix characteristics.
- Gather external data from the managed care market in your community and compare it with internal data of patient information.
- By comparing the internal and external data, you can identify the patient base and decide what services to market to the public and managed care environment.
- Determine a realistic budget defining what you plan to spend on marketing each year.
- Implement the plan with your staff or hire a consultant.
- Monitor the marketing of your practice using phantom patient visits and/or patient-satisfaction surveys.
- Establish a health column or article in the local newspaper or magazine for patient education.
- Be visible within the community and on the Internet.

Negotiation: Getting What You Need

8

Barbara L. Kennedy

The APN and the role of negotiator: What do you need to know?

APNs often find themselves in the role of negotiator. The negotiation process is often filled with common mistakes and misconceptions. This chapter offers suggestions for APNs on how to negotiate and deal with those whom you sense are not negotiating in good faith. Negotiation is both a skill and a process, something that can be successfully learned and applied. Negotiation skills are not instinctive, but, once learned, they can be useful in any circumstance in life. The underlying fundamentals and principles of negotiation remain constant throughout any situation; only the external specifics change. Understanding and applying the basic underlying principles of the negotiation process will provide an excellent foundation for managing your practice. However, it is always important to keep in mind that learning the art of negotiation is a lifelong process.

Where do you begin?

One of the main rules in negotiating is to always negotiate for what you want, but absolutely negotiate for what you need. This, of course, assumes that you, the negotiator, are clear about the difference between what you want and what you must have. This understanding will enable you to know how, when, and if compromise is possible.

When we think of negotiation, the mere word sends waves of panic through most of us. Images of diplomatic peace talks or heated union actions typically come to mind. We may think of negotiation as a set of high-level skills applied mostly to serious matters. The process intimidates many people. We feel that we may be perceived as aggressive or selfish.

Successful negotiation involves skills we use everyday. These are skills we employ when we interact with family, friends, colleagues, and others who we encounter in our daily lives. Even so, otherwise intelligent and highly capable APNs often freeze when they are required to negotiate in a professional capacity. It brings up all sorts of anxieties. In all honesty, there is a legitimate reason for this: Negotiation implies there is or will be conflict.

Conflict, personal or professional, creates discomfort in almost everyone. But think about it. How could we ever have agreement if we did not have conflict first? In a paradoxical kind of way, it is conflict that provides us with the opportunity to come together to agree about something. Conflict takes on a whole new meaning when it is put in that context. APNs historically have not had a lot of experience in resolving conflict through the negotiation process. Typically, they avoid it if possible. Therefore, they have not developed these skills as a component of their professional preparation. However, in this era of rapidly changing employment situations, it has never been more critical for an APN to embrace, and excel at, the role of the negotiator.

It is worth taking some time to evaluate your own feelings and experiences with conflict and negotiation. You must become aware of where your strengths and weaknesses lie in order to enhance and improve your negotiating skills. If you do not know or identify your areas of weakness, be aware that your negotiating counterpart might then use them to your disadvantage. You must also be able to identify your own financial, ethical, and moral bottom line. Without this knowledge of self, you will not be able to know if compromise, or to what degree, is possible.

Whether or not we like it, learning to negotiate wisely is something we must learn to do as professionals. Negotiation is a skill that APNs will need more and more in order to continue to practice successfully in the new millennium.

The skill of negotiation: How can you become a good negotiator?

It is helpful to remember that, like most things, successful negotiation is a set of skills that can be learned. As APNs, we teach our clients everyday. We excel at teaching. We excel at finding learning resources. We excel at identifying personal barriers to growth and learning. We excel at understanding human nature. We excel at active listening and problem solving. We excel at meeting the needs of others. So, with all these skills, APNs should be able to easily learn about negotiation, the negotiating process, and how to ultimately get what they want and need for their profession, clients, and selves. There is nothing unprofessional about getting something for yourself.

Currently, many excellent books (see page 92), tapes, courses, and videos are available about becoming a great negotiator. There are many styles of negotiation. The *win-win* and *interest-based bargaining* styles are two examples. Visit your local or online bookstore in either the self-help or business section to see the variety of tools and techniques that are available. If anything interests you, add it to your professional library. The more you know, the better negotiator you will become. Remember, the basic foundations and principles of negotiation are constant. Books will assist in offering tips on what to do with specific given circumstances. Find an author or style that merges well with your own personal ideas and values.

Another strategy is to seek out advice from people you have seen be successful in negotiations. Find people who are different, as well as like you, in their professional styles of communication. Ask them which techniques work and which do not, and for tips in negotiating that have helped them. If possible, go to union meetings or public hearings. Seek out as many opportunities as possible to watch negotiators at work. There are many styles and subtleties to learn. The world of negotiation is an art with its own rules, culture, and protocols.

Why do you need to become a good negotiator anyway?

Why do you need to be a good negotiator? The answer is simple. As APNs, we are constantly in the process of negotiation. We negotiate with the members of the collaborative health care team. We negotiate with our peers and community support network. We negotiate with our supervisors, employees, and coworkers. We negotiate with our clients. We negotiate with the administration. We negotiate personal and company contracts with local and state governments, schools, Health Maintenance Organizations (HMOs), and other health care institutions. We negotiate with those involved with the structure of our business such as bankers, attorneys, accountants, salespeople, and insurance companies. Without good negotiating skills, managing and maintaining a successful career and business is virtually impossible.

In today's business arena, many APNs are starting their own businesses or subcontracting their services. They are running corporations and clinics. The multiple uses of and the need for negotiating skills are everywhere. So before you begin the process, the first basic piece of information you need to determine is if the organization or individual you are negotiating with is a public-, private-, or community-based concern. This actually makes a very big difference as the strategies you will employ might be vastly different. Don't forget—the underlying principles of good negotiation will remain the same, but the external strategies may change.

The next important piece of information you must have in order to succeed in the negotiating process is knowledge of the players. Know with whom you are negotiating. Know them professionally and, if possible, personally. Know what they like and what their negotiating style is. Know what issues they are likely to be flexible on and on what issues they will be less likely to compromise. This step requires a lot of homework, but the payoff will be well worth the effort. You should do your homework prior to beginning negotiations.

This preparation can take a lot of time, but it is well worth it in the long run. Do you know, for example, which person or persons hold the power to make the final decision concerning your negotiations? Is it the person you are negotiating with or someone else? What does the person look for in an employee or business partner? With this knowledge, you can put your very best face forward and can impact your success in the negotiating process immensely.

Be absolutely sure you know what the 5-year plan is for the venture you are hoping to join or work in partnership with. Are their goals realistic? Is there a potential for growth? How can your service, business, or skill fit into exactly what they need? Research what unique niche you can fill and negotiate for it. Research what the market will bear in terms of cost. If you do not know ahead of time how much an APN is making for a similar service, how will you know if they are offering you or your company a good deal? If you are offering a service, what is the going rate? Know as many details as possible. Negotiators who come into meetings prepared come across with an aura of confidence and that confidence will be respected. Your preparedness also shows that you are genuinely interested in pursuing this opportunity. This then becomes another item in your favor.

Also, be sure you have talked with other employees or contractors prior to your meeting. This information will help you ascertain if the person or company you will be negotiating with has a history of keeping their agreements or negotiating in good faith.

When your verbal negotiation is completed, make sure you do the following:

- Always get whatever you negotiate in writing as soon as possible, even to the smallest detail. Agreements that are not written are soon forgotten.
- Read the contract.

If any corrections, changes, or amendments to the contract have been made, look at the specific section. However, do not only reread those parts that were being corrected; read the *whole* contract again. It is not uncommon to find that an unscrupulous businessperson has changed a different part of the contract hoping you will not take the time to review it again. Despite this deliberate deception, you will be bound to the contract you signed. Whether it is for the private or public sector, always read and reread the final contract. You should not be expected to sign a contract on good faith immediately in the office. If you are pressured to do so, this is a red flag. A reputable counterpart will have no problem with you taking a day or so to review the document thoroughly.

A few basic concepts in negotiation

These basic concepts of negotiation apply to both types of situations—the public and private employer:

- Do not expect to complete an immediate agreement. Negotiation is more frequently a process of incremental steps toward a middle ground.
- Do not be afraid to hear no. No just means no. It doesn't mean they will not say yes to another proposal or even yes to the same offer at a later date.
- It is not personal; it is business.
- Ultimately, if you can't agree, it is okay to disagree.
- Did I mention it is not personal?

There are some essential basic skills that you should always bring to the negotiating table. These include the following:

- Be open minded.
- Actively listen.
- Do your homework prior to getting to the negotiating table, as discussed previously.
- Know the opposition, as discussed previously.
- Keep the process moving. If you come to a roadblock at one issue, move on to the next.
- Build trust by being honest and reliable.
- Know ahead of time what your bottom line is—financially and otherwise.
- Know what is and is not negotiable.
- Know the mission statement and philosophy of your employer, and ensure that what they are offering and discussing is in harmony with these and your values.
- Always keep your word.

Once you have mastered the basics, you can bring other skills to the negotiating table:

- Listen for what you agree on, not just what you don't agree on.
- Contribute out-of-the-box thinking. Look beyond the given parameters.
- Be patient. (Yes, it's hard, but delaying immediate gratification may yield a bigger and more desired agreement in the future.)
- Be aware of your own negotiation style and how to adapt it to the current negotiation. Without flexibility, you will be doomed.
- You do not always need to act quickly, but you must always act decisively.
- Use whatever negotiating techniques you have in your arsenal as long as they do not compromise your values or professional ethics.

In contrast, the following are some actions and behaviors you should *never* bring to the negotiating table:

- Do not get personal. Remember, this is not personal; it is business. Stick to the topic and speak only to the issues at hand.
- Do not make personal attacks on your counterpart's character, history, or career (even if what you have to say is true).
- Do not ask for substantially more than you really want.
- Do not come to the negotiation unprepared and unaware of your bottom line. You must do your homework prior to getting to the negotiating table.
- Do not lose your temper, cry, or yell, unless you are in the big leagues and have woven this action into an artfully brilliant plan. For the rest of us, these behaviors are absolutely forbidden.
- Do not shame or embarrass your counterpart. Again, just stick to the issues.
- Do not argue just for the sake of arguing. If it is not an essential point, drop it.
- Do not let them make you feel guilty. (If they are good, they will use this trick.)
- Do not believe they have your best interests at heart (they rarely do), but negotiate as if they did.
- Never agree to anything that you are not proud of or would not be willing to see on the front page of your local newspaper.

- Never say never as all things are relative. An unacceptable offer in one situation may be appropriate and acceptable in another context.
- Never compromise your values.

In addition to these skills, a really effective negotiator always uses plain common sense. Here are a few ideas worth mentioning no matter how obvious they are:

- Do not be afraid to ask for help.
- Find and use a mentor.
- Talk to someone who has already gone through a process similar to the one you are about to enter.
- Be patient with yourself and remember that for the vast majority of us, negotiating is a new skill.
- Delegate pieces of the negotiating process if appropriate.
- Do not feel you need to go alone. There is no rule that says you cannot bring someone with you.
- Know that there is a difference between the professional and business models. Know the model mindset of your negotiating counterpart.
- Negotiate on the issues, not on how they relate to a particular individual. He or she may be gone tomorrow.
- Understand the concept and importance of "saving face." Learn how to let your counterpart save face without compromising your integrity or values.
- Believe in what you are negotiating for.

Types of Negotiation: Negotiating in the For-profit Sector

The most important thing to remember about the for-profit sector is that its goal is to make money, and as the expression goes, "time is money." Therefore, the negotiation process will likely be faster. This premise is pretty straightforward and understandable. If someone is not working, the company, clinic, office, and so on is not making money—period.

Another factor in private/for-profit business negotiation is that CEOs and/or owners are not legally required to disclose any financial information about the company. For example, they do not need to disclose to you how much they are willing to spend for the pay and/or benefits you are seeking. They do not need to disclose the financial status of the business by opening their books for public inspection (except in very rare cases). They do not need to tell you how much money is at stake, or what other employees are earning or have recently negotiated for.

They will tell you what they are offering, or you will tell them what you are asking for, and this is where the negotiation process will begin. One rule of thumb is discussed in many books on negotiation: It is better to let the other party put their cards on the table first, if possible.

Remember that the for-profit negotiation goal is to make money and get the best value for as few of their dollars as possible. Therefore, you must convince them that you are as valuable as the salary/benefits or working conditions you are seeking. To accomplish this, your personal negotiating skills must be very strong. You will be going it alone. In this situation, it is important to keep a few things in mind:

- Your demands are not visible to the public, so you will have little public support for your issues (if you are negotiating with a large union, that is a different matter that will be discussed later).
- Negotiations are behind closed doors and private. Personal negotiations go on everyday and you are no wiser unless you are the person involved.

As a word of warning, it should also be noted that there should never be any sense of permanent employment status as far as your for-profit employer goes. Be happy with what you have negotiated for, as disgruntled workers are not tolerated long by private employers. If you are not happy, it is best you look for another position. Also, in the private sector, do not openly discuss the outcomes of your negotiation settlement. Private negotiations are meant to be just that—private.

Examples of for-profit situations that the APN will encounter include, but are by no means limited to, the following:

- Private health care offices
- Private hospitals

- Private schools for academic or nursing services
- Private colleges and universities for academic or nursing services
- Independent consulting work
- Expert witness or case reviewer for legal matters
- Religious institutions

Types of Negotiation: Negotiating in the Public Sector

In contrast, if you are going to be negotiating with an employer who is in the public sector such as a governmental agency, state university system, government-run clinic, and so on, the approach will be substantially different. This is mainly because very little of the negotiation process is *not* public knowledge. Everyone knows what the issues are and just how much money is on the table for negotiation. It is part of the public record. The only thing to be negotiated is how and by whose interpretation the legislative intent is to be enacted. For good or for ill, this makes a negotiator in this situation very visible to the public because very little of his or her position and demands is not public. It is also part of the public record.

You must remember that when a governmental agency is involved, there is an implication that somehow the public good is being addressed. So the public ultimately has a right to know how and where their money has been spent. And, although those involved also do not have permanent status, because they are working in the field of public service, both administrators and employees have the freedom to be more outspoken. To this end, these employees are most often represented by a labor union of some type. And, for reasons not covered in this chapter, the process of negotiating settlements can take longer.

The following are some examples of public concerns that the APN might face:

- State, county, or local governmental agencies
- Federal government such as the Veterans Administration
- Public health clinics
- Public state or county colleges and universities

Working in unions: The private or public sector

Perhaps you will find that you have risen or are pushed to a leadership position in your employee union. APNs are rarely in this situation, as most APN positions tend to be professional, nonunion positions. However, should you find that this is the case, here are a few tips:

- In most unionized business, there will be a dominant union.
- If your group is not already attached to this dominant union, try to become a local unit if possible.
- Negotiate as follows: "We will accept what is offered to the (larger) union."
- Let the larger, more powerful dominant union be the pattern setter.
- Let the administration settle with the dominant union first.

If the powers that be are aware of your affiliation and alliance with the larger union, they are more likely to address your demands with greater deference. Keep in mind that when your group has allied with the larger union, you will be expected, if not required, to support its actions including strikes.

Negotiating as a partner

A partnership is an interesting and often successful type of business. It offers the participant the hands-on contact and control without all the responsibility. You can actually take a weekend off! However, we have all heard people say, "never go into business with your family or friends." There is good reason for this. Remember, negotiation and the decisions that need to be negotiated are not personal; they are business. In our personal lives, it is very hard to keep the two separated.

Be that as it may, you should consider a few items prior to entering into a partnership:

- How well do you know this person or company?
- How long have you known them and what is their history?
- What is their reputation?

- Are their values and goals in harmony with your own?
- What will you gain from this partnership?
- What will you have to give up for this partnership?
- Do the benefits outweigh the risks?
- Will this partnership benefit them more than you?

When and if you decide to go into a partnership, all aspects must be negotiated including issues such as how the partnership will be dissolved if necessary. This is rarely something anyone wants to think about, but remember, this is business, not personal. Get every detail in writing and read the contract prior to signing it to ensure it is what you negotiated for.

Negotiating as a subcontractor

This section does not need to address many issues concerned with negotiation itself. The principles that apply elsewhere apply here as well. Negotiating a subcontractor's position either for yourself or your company requires the preparedness that we spoke about in a previous section. Know that as a subcontractor, you will be required to sign a binding contract so if you have grossly underestimated your costs, you will be stuck with it, possibly for a very long time. Part of your preparedness is understanding the market and the price it will bear. As you are the employer, you will be responsible for all your state, local, and federal taxes. Determining costs such as worker's compensation, disability, liability insurance, vacation, health care benefits, and so on will depend on whether you are going solo or have employees. Employee benefits alone can be anywhere in the range of 20% to 30% above the employee's salary. For the purposes of this chapter, let us only say that you must be well informed to negotiate a workable contract.

Negotiating with employees and negotiating when you are in a position of power

This is by far the simplest form of negotiation as generally you will be in a position of power. Although all the fundamentals still apply, negotiating from a position of power has a very simple formula:

- Treat others as you would like to be treated.
- Be fair, honest, and consistent.
- Give what you can, not what you can get away with.

Your employees will thank you. This is generally reflected in a long-term, hardworking, and loyal member of your team.

Negotiating when you are not in a position of power

Despite your best intentions and thorough preparation, you may find yourself in a position where you have little or no real power. Needless to say, this is a very frustrating situation to be in. Despite all your merit and excellence as a negotiator, you have no real means of securing what you want. Many professionals find themselves in this situation and all too frequently spend an extreme amount of energy and frustration trying to change the inevitable. The following are a few concepts and insights to keep in mind:

- That's how it is. Accept it and deal with it. If you can't deal with it, move on.
- Do not compromise your values, even at an uneven table. Consider whether you want to work for anyone who would make you compromise your values anyway. If you cannot leave immediately, plan to do so as soon as possible.
- Remember that the reasons and agendas for being at the negotiating table may be different.
- Just because you negotiated does not mean the outcome is fair or just. Frequently, there is an imbalance of power and the dominant voice will be heard regardless of the issues.
- Without your knowledge, the agenda or outcome may already be signed, sealed, and delivered before you even get to the negotiating table. If this happens to you, figure out how it happened and do everything possible to not let it happen to you again.

What do you do if after a great amount of effort you still feel that you cannot engage in the negotiating process successfully?

Sometimes, despite our best efforts, we can't acquire the level of expertise we feel we need. Occasionally, an issue arises that needs to be negotiated before you have had time to acquire good negotiating skills. Here is a tip: Take someone with you who can negotiate. Let that person speak and act on your behalf. You will be there to give the ultimate thumbs up or thumbs down.

Frequently, we are better at negotiating on behalf of someone else than we are for ourselves. If this is true for you, follow this advice, at least for the time being.

What do you do if you smell a rat?

What do you do if you feel that your counterparts are not being honest with you? What do you do if you get the feeling that they are trying to pull a fast one that you will live to regret? These, unfortunately, are pragmatic questions. One solution, if you have the luxury of time, is to negotiate in good faith on an issue that you are not particularly attached to the outcome of as a test. See what the response is the first time you exercise your negotiated rights. If the feedback you receive is negative, you've got a rat. The person will have demonstrated that he or she cannot be trusted to negotiate in good faith. If you absolutely must stay in this professional situation, do so with your eyes wide open. However, the best advice that you can receive is to start looking for another position with an individual or corporation whose mission and philosophy match their actions and your needs. Find a situation where the words of your contract are worth more than the paper they are written on.

Mutual trust and respect are essential components to any professional relationship. There is no reason to work without them:

- Remember the saying, "a leopard does not change its spots."
- Do not be fooled into a false sense of security when the fair weather arrives. If you have identified a rat, he or she will still be a rat tomorrow.

- Rats lie. Rats do not view lying as lying. They view their statement as a necessary means to facilitate their immediate need. In the rat world, the means, any means, justify the end. They will think you an idealistic fool if you do not share this view.
- Do not trust the identified rat again.
- If you must work with the rat, have nothing more than a superficial relationship. Keep your relationship polite and always professional.

What about issues of gender?

Approximately 97% of nurses are female. This obviously leads us to discuss the specific issues of women in the workplace and women as negotiators. Suffice it to say that the issues are complicated. Women's roles and the role of nurses have changed drastically since the inception of the APN in the 1960s. Women still face many challenges in the workplace. There is sufficient evidence to prove that the glass-ceiling phenomenon exists. Whether or not it is true will not be debated here. What needs to be addressed is the question of whether negotiating as a woman is a different skill. If so, how is it different? Here are some thoughts to consider:

- If you believe the glass ceiling exists where you are working, do not address it. Stick to the issues. Negotiate in good faith. If after a reasonable amount of time you have evidence that gender barriers still remain, move on to a work environment where they do not.
- You do not need to behave like anyone else to be a good negotiator. Be yourself.
- Remember that you have been negotiating all your life—you are good at this.
- There are many examples of strong, effective women negotiators. Learn about them and study what has made them successful.
- Remember that times change. Negotiation styles change. Stay current with business trends.

- If you sense that you are being negotiated with as a woman rather than as a professional, make your counterpart aware that this is unacceptable.

The world of negotiation: Respecting the process

Finally, the world of negotiation has its own values and culture. Whether or not you believe this to be the case, it is—live with it. In your negotiations, do not spend any time trying to fix or rail against the system. That is not your goal. That is another goal for another time, if you are so inclined. Concentrate on your current negotiating objectives and respect the process.

You should follow and respect the protocols of negotiation. Whether or not you feel it is worthwhile, go through the motions. Learn the language. Observe the protocols. Experienced negotiators will treat you and your issues with much more respect and consideration if you do. Do not go into a negotiating situation being ignorant of the process. If you do this with an experienced negotiator as your adversary, you have sealed your fate.

After things are all said and done, the negotiations may not go the way you had hoped. Remember to always leave the negotiation table with

- Your self-respect.
- A willingness to try something new.
- Your integrity and values intact.

If you act with such principles, it is highly reasonable to predict that you will be a successful negotiator, a valued colleague, and a professional in the best sense of the word.

Effective Leadership in Practice Management

9

Ann Glasgow

Why should APNs know about leadership roles in the management of a practice?

APNs are faced with multiple challenges and changes within a clinical practice that require leadership and pertinent management functions. To successfully manage a practice and be responsive to ever changing practice needs and maintain a central role in the delivery of health care, APNs consciously develop leadership characteristics. In doing so, APNs soon discover innovative pathways to direct quality care, and health promotion, prevention, and restoration.

In order to cultivate the attributes necessary to become a successful leader and manager, APNs are faced with the continuing challenge of accumulating knowledge through education and experience. Specific skills require a steady upward progression through the novice-advanced-beginner-competent-proficient-expert continuum. With the emergence of APNs into independent practice settings, progress in the development of these skills can be advanced with strong self-esteem and a self-nurturing system that fosters role socialization.

What strategies are used to develop leadership and management skills?

As an APN, the most important element in success is the development of strong self-esteem and a healthy sense of self. Here are some pertinent self-nurturing strategies that promote a commitment to developing your personal self:

- Have a vision.
- Develop your life blueprint.
- Embrace positive life strategies.
- Be assertive.
- Surround yourself with nurturing family, friends, and colleagues.
- Take care of yourself.
- Seek a daily haven for a peaceful escape.
- Learn to say no without guilt.
- Learn to let go.
- Deal with anger constructively.

Role socialization is a continuous process that empowers the APN with characteristic leadership and management skills. To facilitate the development of these attributes, the following strategies may be utilized:

- Conduct an organizational analysis of the practice setting.
- Define position descriptions to guide practice performance.
- Continually articulate, clarify, and revise your advanced practice role to patients, families, colleagues, and the public.
- Generate a monthly activity summary.
- Conduct a periodic self-assessment of your development in the advanced practice role.
- Use personal planning skills.
- Use your imagination and take risks.
- Develop yearly, measurable objectives, including an implementation and evaluation plan.
- Identify a suitable mentor who is trustworthy, nurturing, accessible, ambitious, influential, and knowledgeable, and with whom it is easy to communicate.
- Cultivate supportive collegial relationships.
- Keep the ambiguities of your practice setting in perspective and maintain your sense of humor.
- Maintain a positive self-concept.
- Trust your own intuitive feelings.

- Nurture yourself without feeling guilty or selfish.
- Pace yourself for the long haul.
- Maintain your commitment to lifelong learning.
- Keep abreast of local, regional, and national legislative, regulatory, and health policy issues.

What are the differences in leadership and management?

Although leadership and management roles are different, they are intertwined within an APN practice. Leadership can be defined as the process of influencing others. Management expands this to include the planning, organizing, motivating, and controlling stages to achieve the desired outcome. For an optimal relationship to exist between these two concepts, an APN's practice should demonstrate the integration of leadership and good management characteristics.

What are the essentials of successful leadership?

An APN's clinical and professional leadership is based on expertise derived from education and clinical experience. Effective leadership characteristics are linked to the personal mastery of skills, intuition, self-understanding, value congruency, vision, risk taking, mentoring, and empowerment. The following characteristics are emphasized as core leadership qualities:

- **Intelligence.**   Knowledge, judgment, decisiveness, achievement, ambition, sound analytical and problem-solving skills, and oral fluency
- **Personality.**   Adaptability, creativity, innovation, cooperation, alertness, self-confidence, personal integrity, emotional balance and control, nonconformity, independence, and dedication to one's job
- **Ability.**   The ability to enlist cooperation, interpersonal skills, tact, diplomacy, prestige, and social participation, and to learn from adversity

What are the basic leadership styles?

Leadership style is best defined as how the leader relates to members of the group at work. The following leadership styles are characterized according to relevant behaviors exhibited by the leader:

- Charismatic leadership
  - ➤ Develops an emotional relationship between the leader and group.
  - ➤ Arouses strong feelings of loyalty and enthusiasm from the group.
  - ➤ The leader communicates the plan to which the group adheres.
- Authoritarian leadership
  - ➤ Provides little freedom—the group is incapable of making decisions.
  - ➤ The leader determines policies, giving orders and direction to the group.
  - ➤ Minimal openness and trust exist between the leader and group.
  - ➤ Procedures are well defined, activities are predictable, and the group is secure.
  - ➤ High productivity, good quality, and very efficient.
  - ➤ Communication flows downward.
  - ➤ Criticism is punitive.
- Democratic leadership
  - ➤ Provides moderate freedom—the group is capable of achieving goals.
  - ➤ The leader acts as facilitator, actively guiding the group toward the goal.
  - ➤ The leader provides constructive criticism, offers information, makes suggestions, and asks pertinent questions.
  - ➤ Involves shared responsibility in achieving goals.
  - ➤ Less efficient, but fosters more self-motivation and creativity.
  - ➤ High quality.
  - ➤ Communication flows up and down.
- Laissez-faire leadership
  - ➤ Provides much freedom with minimal control.

➤ Motivates by support when requested.
➤ Minimal involvement of the leader.
➤ Decision making is done by the group.
➤ Emphasis is on the group with the abdication of leader responsibility.
➤ Criticism is not given.
➤ Variable quality due to inefficiency.
➤ Communication exists between members of the group, upward and downward.

• Situational leadership
➤ The level of direction is linked to the level of group maturity.
➤ Directive style—giving clear instruction and specific directions to an immature group.
➤ Coaching style—two-way communication helps a maturing group gain confidence and motivation.
➤ Supporting style—active two-way communication with a mature group enhances the use of their talents.
➤ Delegating—a highly mature group is given responsibilities for planning and decision making.
➤ Focuses on the accomplishment of tasks and interpersonal relationships between the leader and group.

• Transactional leadership
➤ Focuses on management tasks.
➤ The leader is a caretaker.
➤ Uses trade-offs to meet goals.
➤ Has unidentified shared values.
➤ Examines causes.

• Transformational leadership
➤ Identifies common values.
➤ The leader is committed.
➤ Inspires others with vision.
➤ Has a long-term vision.
➤ Looks at effects.
➤ Empowers others.

Becoming an effective leader is a continuous process of identifying and managing one's personal and professional boundaries. The essence of leadership development requires the practice of applicable leadership styles to experience the components of management and associated outcomes. Over time, APNs feel secure in their type of practice leadership. The caring leadership style, prevalent in health care, is an expansion of transformational leadership. APNs moving into an independent practice possess an integration of caring leadership characteristics and management functions—the key qualities of an entrepreneur.

Effective leadership requires an understanding of the needs and goals that motivate people, the knowledge to apply leadership skills, and the interpersonal skills to influence others. The following are strategies for actively acquiring an entrepreneurial leadership style that creates an environment that is stimulating, motivating, and empowering:

- Accept responsibility.
- Talk less and listen more—encourage communication and the sharing of ideas and information.
- Recognize the expertise of others.
- Foster an atmosphere of collegiality and mutual trust.
- Always give before you get—give colleagues and staff a reason for doing whatever it is you ask of them.
- Foster creativity, independence, and professional growth.
- Work on ways to improve a situation or solve a problem. Do not condemn, criticize, or complain.
- Always greet others with a positive, affirmative statement.
- Praise or positively recognize staff and colleagues.
- Work on discovering individual group members' unique personal and professional needs.
- Remember the names of the people you work with.
- Write informal appreciation notes to show appreciation and reinforce positive performance.
- Think, act, and look successful.
- Always think good thoughts about yourself and others.
- Smile often—it generates enthusiasm and goodwill.
- Get out of the office—make a point to circulate among those who work in your circle of influence.

What tools are essential for the leader in a management position to solve problems?

The leader/manager who uses analytical tools that give order and direction to the resolution of decisions makes decision making that much easier:

- Decision grids enable the manager to list alternatives and examine financial, political, departmental, and practice effects.
- Decision trees allow the visualization of outcomes with actions taken.
- Program Evaluation and Review Technique (PERT) determines the timing of decisions in a flowchart format that keeps everyone abreast with early problem identification.

These techniques are useful, but not foolproof to the human element of management and leadership.

What are the primary obstacles when APNs become entrepreneurs?

Two primary obstacles prevent APNs from achieving the entrepreneurial vision in a clinical and professional practice.

The Star Complex

In this situation, an APN's boundary management of him- or herself as an APN is lost. The APN may be thinking of him- or herself as a "wannabee." APNs are vulnerable to being seduced into believing they are more than a nurse. The strategy for managing this obstacle is effective mentoring by a powerful APN with an intact nursing identity. Essential to resolving this issue is the use of clear and concise communication skills, which provide an appropriate response to colleagues and disbelieving others.

Unity Versus Fragmentation

This obstacle to leadership involves an APN's tendency to separate and establish boundaries that distinguish him or her from one another, thereby blocking opportunities for the increased power that unity brings. The following guidelines help move from fragmentation toward unity:

- Direct disciplined attention to the issue of unity.
- Translate the goal of unification into a shared vision.
- Develop a forum of providers and educators to explore, identify, and regulate stress related to merging boundaries previously viewed as impenetrable.
- Listen with respect to leadership voices.
- Return to the referent professional association for continuing dialogue and support of outcomes from the forum.
- Emerge from the systematic exploration of unity with a clear goal of support for the continued development of the APN leadership role.

Does empowerment play a part in the leadership and management of an APN practice?

Empowerment can be defined as an activity directed to increasing people's control over their lives. It enables people to recognize and feel their strengths, abilities, and personal power through an increased knowledge, control, and command of resources. For the APN to survive the ever-changing health care system, it is essential to include these points:

- An understanding of knowledge that fuels commitment to a program of continuous improvement in health service delivery
- The skills to apply the four areas of improvement knowledge: systems theories, variation theories, psychological theories, and learning theories
- The ability to integrate the work of health professionals to meet individual and community health needs
- A professional ethic that supports such integrated work

The empowerment continuum is influenced by the evolving role of women, societal changes that increase people's involvement in decision-making processes, increases in educational levels, and economic factors.

The following are components of empowerment that APNs use to assess where they find themselves in the continuum for their practice:

- **Context.**   Establishes the vision that fosters unity and sets the pivotal point of the decision-making process.
- **Structure.**   Organizational structures dictate the hierarchical levels with centralized control of authority and decision making, which can facilitate or impede the process.
- **Process.**   Creates a reflective process of inquiry in the APN practice.

As the role of the APN emerges within the health care delivery system, empowerment is an integral component for successful leadership and management. Increasing political awareness and involvement with refined skills from continuous knowledge acquisition equips the APN with essential elements for practice success.

Skills for empowerment include a continuous use of refined knowledge, the ability to understand and communicate, the ability to plan appropriate actions and proceed with necessary steps to achieve a goal, the ability to arrive at alternate solutions, implementation, and the ability to delegate to others. To foster a positive practice outcome from delegating to others, you should incorporate the following:

- Provide a clear understanding of the desired results.
- Give a clear sense of the level of initiative your staff can enjoy. Must they wait until told, seek permission, make recommendations, act and report immediately, or act and report periodically?
- Clarify assumptions up front.
- Provide people who are assigned work with as much time, resources, and access to you as is needed.
- Set a time and place for presenting and reviewing the results of completed work.
- Never accept uncompleted work. Completed work gives responsibility to the staff while increasing their ability to respond wisely in different situations.

The concept of empowerment is also applicable to the patient. The trend now is to include patients in the decision-making process so they become active participants in health promotion, prevention, and restoration. Enabling patients with their own power and control of life promotes better adherence to the plan of care, which yields a more positive outcome. APNs delegate effectively to those equipped with specific abilities to achieve an established vision. This permits the entrepreneur to seek additional avenues and resources to accomplish even greater visions. Sharing responsibility with those in the work force or with patients empowers APNs to become a vital component in achieving established goals.

An APN who is a risk taker and willing to let go and become an entrepreneur should focus on this key concept of empowering others for more positive outcomes. Several small books with many of the attributes found in entrepreneurs take only a few hours to read. The information is a goldmine:

- *Who Moved My Cheese?* by Spencer Johnson
- *Fish* by Stephen C. Lundin
- *Getting to Yes* by Roger Fisher, William Ury, and Bruce Patton
- *Virtues of Leadership* by William J. Bennett
- *Blueprint for Life* by Casey Treat
- *Life Strategies* by Phillip C. McGraw
- *Beyond Winning* by Robert H. Mnookin
- *It Takes More Than a Carrot and a Stick* by Wess Roberts
- *How to Make People Like You* by Nicholas Boothman
- *The One Minute Manager* by Kenneth Blanchard and Spencer Johnson
- *Please Don't Just Do What I Tell You!* by Bob Nelson
- *Winnie-the-Pooh on Management* by Roger E. Allen
- *Manager's Handbook* by Robert Heller
- *Power* by Robert Greene

Do you possess the necessary leadership qualities?

Many qualities needed to become a successful leader have been discussed in this chapter. Do you possess leadership qualities? Do a quick assessment of yourself. Find those qualities that need polishing and strive to become the entrepreneur within. (See Appendix 4 for a leadership self-assessment text.)

Collaborative APN Practice

10

Andrea Wolf

What is collaborative practice?

Although collaboration between professionals of different disciplines occurs at all levels, the discussion of collaborative practice in this case is limited to relationships between APNs and physicians:

- *Collaborative practice* is a joint effort between an APN and a physician for the purpose of sharing expertise to achieve optimal patient care.
- The collaboration between APNs and physicians requires cooperation in which each professional contributes a unique set of skills.
- The collaboration among APNs and physicians is different from the supervision of an APN practice by a physician who controls the decision-making capacity of the APN.
- Collaborative practice need not be defined by the employment arrangement chosen by the APN. An APN in an independent private practice may form a collaborative practice agreement with a physician that determines the relationship between the APN and the physician.

What are the critical elements of true collaborative practice?

- First, collaborative practice requires competence on the part of each member of the collaborative team. Competence is achieved through the appropriate education and clinical experience. The

93

APN must have a graduate degree and be nationally certified in a given specialty.

- Collaborative practice requires the establishment of equal authority between the physician and APN in a work setting. Responsibilities are shared. Collegiality between professionals will foster the mutual trust that needs to be established to allow shared authority. In this manner, the relationship between physician and nurse is collaborative rather than supervisory.
- Communication must be open and dynamic. This allows a flexible shift in responsibility and decision making between professionals when patient care requires a particular type of expertise.
- In collaborative practice, each professional must be confident in the skills he or she possesses and be assertive when patient care requires it. A lack of assertiveness is detrimental in the care of the patient. Input from each appropriate professional is imperative. The ability of professionals to be assertive and able to handle emotions when conflict arises avoids counterproductive interaction.

What are the advantages of collaborative practice?

- Collaborative practice improves patient outcomes while enhancing personal professional satisfaction.
- Collaboration improves access to care and reduces health care costs by utilizing manpower resources.
- Collaborative practice with improved communication between professionals enhances mutual trust and respect.

Are there different models of collaborative practice?

Different models for collaborative practice are used, depending on the APN's background and the setting in which care is provided:

- The APN sees a patient, regardless of the rapidity of the onset of an illness or complexity, and provides ongoing care, collaborating with physicians when necessary. The APN decides when the physician's opinion is needed. (The physician might never see the patient.) If the patient becomes medically unstable, the APN and physician share patient management to provide the best possible care. The APN will continue to expand his or her knowledge and skills through continued experiences with complex medical problems.

- The APN working in a private practice frequently sees a subset of practice patients. For example, he or she may see less complex, healthier patients with acute primary care problems. Or the APN may see stable chronic patients, such as those with diabetes and hypertension, who require a lot of patient education. If a patient becomes medically unstable, the APN refers the patient to a physician who, at that point, assumes care of the patient. This model for collaboration is considered efficient because it anticipates that the APN will practice independently, requiring less input from the physician. The APN must have the opportunity to increase his or her knowledge and skills in order to expand the scope of the practice.

- The APN performs a history and physical exam, which is then presented to the physician who establishes a plan of care for every patient encounter. This type of collaboration is common in specialty practices where patients (referred from primary care physicians) are seeking consultation with the hope of receiving an expert opinion. This model is used when the patient, the physician referring, or the physician referred to is dismayed if only the APN sees the patient. The APN must present every patient to the physician, even if the physician sees the patient only briefly.

- Patients alternate between seeing the APN and the physician during the course of their ongoing care. This model takes over when Medicare "incident-to" billing is used to show the physician's active participation in the care of the patient.

- The APN working in an acute care setting usually collaborates in the interest of the patient with a variety of professionals, including physicians, respiratory therapists, and dietitians. The APN frequently functions as the coordinator of care during the patient's hospital stay.

- The APN sees the patient for the purpose of providing a particular service. For example, a Clinical Nurse Specialist (CNS) working in an obstetrics/gynecology practice provides pregnancy counseling and education for each prenatal patient. When a problem arises, the CNS immediately refers the patient to the collaborating physician.

What barriers to collaborative practice can APNs expect to encounter?

Historically, the passive, subservient role nurses have found themselves in with physicians has not only formed barriers to effective communication concerning patient care, but also continues to be the largest single impediment in the achievement of a positive present-day nurse-physician collaborative relationship. Gender issues emanating from the old traditional standard need to be addressed if growth is to be achieved. The media's constant portrayal of nurses as subservient to physicians amplifies this negative education. All these constraints, however, are unable to totally hide patient benefits—a healthy outgrowth of new APN-physician collaborative practices! To meet increasing world health challenges, APNs with their collaborative partners look forward to the day when the American Academy of Nurse Practitioners (AANP), the American Nurses Association (ANA), and the American Medical Association (AMA) collaborate on an even playing field based on strong support for each other for the benefit of the patient:

- A central obstacle to effective collaboration is that of turf issues regarding the economics of health care. APNs whose scope of practice overlaps with physicians may encounter resistance in their attempt to establish a collaborative relationship. Physicians who see the APN practice as encroaching upon their domain are often concerned about a loss of revenue. Turf issues are particularly problematic for new APNs who have difficulty articulating their new roles.
- Philosophical differences between the practice of medicine and nursing are a stumbling block in forming collaborative relationships. Opportunities for valuable input in patient situa-

tions, arising from different philosophical perspectives, may be missed when the unique contributions of each profession are not recognized.

- Regulatory issues continue to pose barriers to the effective collaboration between APNs and physicians. States differ in their approach to regulating APN practices. States that use the term *supervision* rather than *collaboration* to describe the relationship between the physician and APN force their APNs to seek supervisory agreements with physicians just to practice as APNs. The interpretation of the regulatory language enables physicians to control an APN practice, thus undermining the requisite of professional autonomy for true collaboration.

- Institutional policies (such as not offering hospital privileges) pose further barriers to APNs practicing in outpatient settings— for example, APNs who want to provide care to their patients who require hospitalization. True collaborative physicians who value the APN's expertise often find themselves powerless to influence the much needed peer and legislative change in policy. This forces physicians who hope to expand their practices by working with APNs for the benefit of their patients to terminate their collaborative agreement.

- Organizational policies pose obstacles to collaboration by discouraging physicians from entering collaborative relationships with APNs. In some states, organized medicine successfully lobbies their state medical board to continue their jurisdiction over APN practice. Enlightened physicians working successfully side by side with APNs are growing in numbers. One day, in the interest of quality patient care, organized medicine will wake up to find itself not only facilitating, but also benefiting from its healthy collaboration with APNs!

How do legislative and regulatory concerns influence collaborative practice?

State rules and regulations dictate the collaborative practice agreements that currently exist between APNs and physicians. For example, in Maryland, an APN cannot practice without a collaborative agreement with a physician who is approved and has filed with the Maryland Board of Nursing, which includes prescriptive privileges. However, in Pennsylvania, the collaborative agreement approved by the Pennsylvania Board of Nursing pertains only to prescriptive privileges. An APN is not required to show proof of a collaborative relationship with a physician, even though the rules and regulations require the APN to have a collaborating physician in order to practice.

Overall, despite the strong opposition from organized medicine, legislative changes in the past decade have enabled APNs to expand their scope of practice by allowing increased autonomy in their delivery of patient care. For example, all states now allow some level of regulatory prescribing authority. (See Appendix 5 for a list of state positions on prescriptive authority for APNs.)

How does managed care influence collaborative practice?

Health care practice in ambulatory settings is influenced more by the emergence of managed care systems than any other single factor. Managed care is seen as an impetus for collaborative practice agreements between APNs and physicians largely because true collaborative practice, by using professionals effectively, results in decreased health care costs. However, reimbursement for APN services may require that certain policies (seen as damaging to the collaborative practice relationship) be in place. For example, rules requiring the supervision of an APN may require the physician to document supervision by cosigning the records of every APN patient encounter. Similar policies appear to stifle an APN practice, especially when policies are more restrictive than the regulatory rules of the state. Practices that have contracts with various managed care systems have difficulty keeping track of which patients belong to a given system. This results in the adoption of restrictive policies that apply to APN patients.

Medicare billing policies, frequently seen as restrictive to APN practice, serve to undermine the collaborative relationship. Incident-to physician care billing requires that services provided by the APN be delivered under the direct supervision of the physician. In order to bill this way, the physician must be in the same building at the time services are delivered and the APN must be employed by the physician. The physician is also required to provide initial service to the patient and see the patient frequently enough to show continued involvement with the patient's care. Since this type of directive is difficult to interpret, it is risky for APNs to bill this way. However, billing under an APN's own number results in a lower level of reimbursement. Practices in which APNs see a large number of Medicare patients may notice a substantial loss of revenue if APNs bill under their own numbers. This not only influences the physician's decisions about collaborative practice relationships, but it also affects the decision of whether to even consider a collaborative practice agreement with an APN.

What settings are appropriate for collaborative practice for APNs?

Opportunities exist in a variety of settings that enable APNs to develop successful collaborative agreements with physicians. The following is a list of settings to consider:

- Primary care practice (e.g., family, pediatric, and obstetrics/gynecology)
- Outpatient specialty practice (e.g., cardiology, gastroenterology, and oncology)
- Long-term care facility
- Home care
- Nursing center
- Inpatient surgical service (e.g., cardiothoracic surgery)
- Hospital residency teaching service

What are the components of a collaborative practice agreement?

The suggested components of a collaborative practice agreement in a primary care setting are outlined as follows:

- The agreement includes a list of definitions describing what collaborative practice means for the particular practice setting, the nature of the collaborative relationship, the job descriptions of the APN and the physician collaborator, and the organizational plan for the practice.

- Clinical issues include considerations such as patient assignment, documentation, diagnostic testing, prescriptive issues, specialty consultations, hospital admissions, and emergency coverage.
- Business or legal issues are included (e.g., start-up costs, the handling of income, reimbursement issues, licensing, credentialing, and malpractice insurance).
- Provisions are made for ongoing evaluation of the agreement.

What are the strategies for a successful collaborative relationship?

Prior to entering the collaborative practice, you should do the following:

- Assess each professional for personal characteristics such as assertiveness, communication skills, competence, and ethics.
- Plan a discussion among practice professionals about philosophies, goals, and the role of each member of the collaborative team.
- Establish the financial reimbursement, the division of responsibilities, and the expected time commitment of each member.
- Develop written guidelines that function as the collaborative practice agreement. Include input from each professional.
- Plan administrative leadership that allows continued support of the collaborative team.
- Form a committee representing each professional for the purpose of discussion and consideration of ongoing issues.
- Investigate legislative issues influencing APN practice (prescriptive privileges), and be certain all professionals understand how issues affect day-to-day practice.

After collaborative practice is in place, you should do the following:

- Create opportunities for a small group to attend continuing education conferences in which each professional is encouraged to contribute his or her expertise.
- Arrange social events to increase interaction in an effort to facilitate effective, positive communication in the work setting.
- Educate patients about the nature of the collaborative relationship, including the roles and responsibilities of each professional in order to facilitate the acceptance of the APN and eliminate confusion. Display literature in the practice setting describing the role and responsibilities of each professional.
- Maintain active participation in legislative activities regarding the scope of practice issues. Ask local representatives to support decisions affecting health care and APN practice.
- Maintain membership in nursing organizations at local, state, and national levels.

What other health professionals comprise interdisciplinary teams for collaborative practice with APNs?

Although this discussion has been limited to the relationships between APNs and their collaborating physicians, it must be noted that in some settings, APNs can collaborate with other nurses and health care professionals. These interdisciplinary teams may consist of members of the nursing staff, social workers, physical therapists, occupational therapists, dietitians, APNs in other specialties, and physician specialists. It is essential that the interdisciplinary team caring for patients with complex medical problems maintain as its focus the delivery of patient-centered care. All members of the team must develop the goals for optimal patient outcomes. Communication between professionals is accomplished through patient rounds and conferences in which team members evaluate and update the patient's plan of care. The documentation of patient care by individual professionals must be readily available to all members of the interdisciplinary team. One team member should coordinate the responsibilities and services of each professional to ensure the efficient use of expertise.

Practice and Information Management

11

Jane Young

What is information management?

Information is the result of your search for knowledge. You either know a subject yourself, or you know where you can find information about it. Consider the amount of daily information generated by your practice. When its accuracy and quality are defined, sorted, and organized (managed, if you will), information has tremendous value and can serve as the basis of evaluations and long-term planning.

In management, raw data information is put into a user-friendly, universal language; however, keep in mind that the information eventually changes as collection methods accommodate to higher standards. The need for accurate data produced in an understandable format in a timely manner is of paramount importance.

What information is needed for a successful practice?

Good APNs are aware that in order to have a successful practice, information garnered through day-to-day operations must be monitored and managed. It is necessary to keep daily track of the following, using periodic reports:

- Management
  - ➢ The aging (current, 30, 60, 90, and 120+ days) of accounts receivable.
  - ➢ The number of claims that are *out to insurance* in each aging account category (current, 30, 60, 90, and 120+ days).

➤ The collection system, which includes the account status (in-house collections or those turned over to a collection agency), totals (in each of the previous categories), and letters (first, second, and third collection letters).

➤ Provider and staff schedules with start and stop times for each day (which includes the time marked out for continuing education, meetings, vacations, or home visits) and empty times saved until the day begins for same-day appointments. It is important to have adequate provider coverage for the patient load (more provider hours on Monday and Friday to cover the heavy load or fewer competing provider hours when a new partner is in the process of building a practice).

➤ Appointment scheduling (the length of appointments is based on the patients' needs; the availability of appointments depends on the patients' schedules and which provider is available).

➤ The system of recalling patients for follow-up as well as periodic visits (i.e., annual exams).

➤ Medical and office supply (and equipment) orders, inventory, and usage.

➤ Accounts payable. What is owed to whom and what is the current account balance, including variable and fixed charges?

➤ The status of electronic claims (sent, holding, pending, and paid).

➤ Mailing labels, letter generation, and word processing.

➤ Payroll processing (which includes keeping track of employee benefits).

➤ Statistical report generation (the illnesses being seen most often, the codes most frequently used, the average charge, and similar items).

➤ The transcription and maintenance of patient records.

• Patients

➤ Patient and family demographic and insurance data (name, address, telephone, and so on).

• Billing

➤ Accurate up-to-date codes for office and hospital visits, diagnoses, and procedures.

> Current charges corresponding to information in the previous item.
> Up-to-date insurance company information (where to send claims).
> Insurance filing and electronic claims processing.
> The management of patient accounts, which includes charges, visits, and payments, as well as insurance status (refusals, payments, and requests for more information).
> The production and mailing of patient statements.

- Providers
  > The number of patients seen by each provider/practice in each day, month, and year.
  > The charges produced by each provider for each day, month, and year.
  > The number of hours that each provider schedules for patients in each day, month, and year. Using the scheduled hours, not just those that are busy, enables you to predict what production will be.
  > Provider profiles (updated license numbers and provider numbers for each insurance company; employer identification numbers and the place of service numbers and codes; and Drug Enforcement Agency [DEA] and Board of Pharmacy certificates).

- Miscellaneous
  > Patient clinical information (medications, prescriptions, chart notes, laboratory and x-ray data, and consultation information).
  > Provider privileges at hospitals.
  > Support staff time in and out.
  > Support staff scheduling.

As the practice owner, what do you want information management to do for you?

Refer to your mission statement. It will help set priorities to determine which of the following is most important to you.

Money In: Production

The knowledge and frustration of knowing that the cost of doing business must be met for the practice to exist is reflected in the saying, "money doesn't talk, it swears." Without money, there is little health care, no services, and no jobs. Continual practice and financial evaluation provides assurance that you will meet your costs plus income in excess of expenses.

Money is like a sixth sense—without it, you can't make use of the other five. It also has a lot in common with life; you can't ignore either fact. Money matters. The productiveness of each provider determines the total practice income available to meet practice expenses. Keep in mind: Time is money.

To measure productiveness, evaluate each provider's contribution (charges) to determine if each person is producing his or her proportionate part of the practice income. Evaluation tells you if the provider's individual production is sufficient to support the anticipated salaries and the rest of the practice expense. Production improvements and maintenance are plainly visible in monthly reports. A clear report enables you to raise valid questions such as the following: Is too much time allotted per patient? Are there periods when everyone seems busy, but the total production is down? What are people doing? Is there an unusually large number of "no-charges" because best friends, neighbors, Cousin Joes, and Aunt Minnies have been in?

Money Management

It is either a thief or a talented business manager who successfully eats his or her dessert before dealing with the vegetables. Hopefully, in your practice, you are working with the manager and consuming the vegetables first. Money is usually appreciated more than poverty. The moral of the story is that although providers supply care, it is imperative that the manager constantly monitor production and income. As a manager, you should ask the following questions:

- Where is your money?
- How many charges out of the total have been properly billed and payment received?

- How many charges have been accepted by your clearinghouse?
- How many charges have successfully reached their destination, i.e., the correct third-party payer?
- How long have insurance companies or patients used a long tongue and a short hand and not paid for the service received?
- How accurately is your coding person coding?
- Is your collector doing an honorable job?
- What is the collection ratio (dollars received in the mail divided by the total dollars collected) for payments received in the mail?
- What is your collection experience at the checkout desk (dollars collected at the desk divided by the total dollars collected)?
- What percentage of the income comes from each insurance company, and what percentage is from managed care?
- Are there different collection rates for different times of the year? (Is it down in the summer due to vacations? Is it down in the beginning of the year due to deductibles?)

Money Out: Expenses

The world is generally in favor of a budget balanced between income and expenses. This is no less true when roaming the fields of health care. It begs the following question: After the produced income is collected, how do you spend it? Your information management system needs to keep track of your vendors, budget, and spending. (Beware of the little expenses; a tiny leak can sink a ship.) Monitoring expenses decreases surprise and enables you to plan future expenditures. Accounts payable information enables you to save for new equipment, staff education, and/or a change of location. At tax time, management information is the core of the apple.

Evaluation

Each evaluation is based on a good system of information. Put simply, a good system of information informs. We are reminded of the chat between an attorney and his client when the attorney volunteered, "I have read your case, Ms. Jones, and I'm no smarter now than when I began," to which Ms. Jones replied, "Possibly not, Mr. Smith, but you are far better informed."

An information management system in its element collects and offers history you will constantly use to evaluate the past and design the future of the practice. Perhaps you want an improved connection with outside laboratories, your own x-ray facilities, or the ability to access diagnostic studies. Do you plan to make Internet services available to your patients? How soon can you offer patient and/or staff education or instruction through your computer system? Will it save time? Consider your options carefully.

How much should you spend on an information system?

In order to determine what you can pay for an information system, review your nursing practice vision, mission, business plan, and desire before arriving at a reasonable balance. Secondly, determine from your budget how much money will be available and by what date. Is it better that a new project be paid outright or leased to become a depreciable business expense? The third step is to establish priorities! What do you want to accomplish and in what order—first, second, third, and so on? The order you choose determines the number of support staff you need. Certain functions of your information system either create or eliminate jobs. Every choice affects your budget. Many functions you have previously done outside the hallowed halls using external contractors are workable in-house, with an information system (coding, patient statements, payroll, and other activities). Conversely, items such as appointment confirmation (done through a computer interface with your phone system) and computer system management may eliminate the need for one staff member. Finally, determine what information must be readily available. The answer determines where you begin. It is important to establish your financial limits *before* you begin spending. Overspending quickly diminishes what little power desire creates.

It's time to get down to business. Recognize that certain aspects of an information management system cost money, regardless of which system you use. Consider the computer system. In addition to the actual hardware and software costs at the time of purchase, the vendor is able to estimate the average annual cost of upkeep and upgrades. The method of upgrading is important. Are upgrades Internet-based and automatic, or do you buy each upgrade? The estimated life of the system before it is obsolete is valuable information for planning the future. The vendor's commitment to maintaining and developing the system lets you know how much you are able to count on them versus how much is your responsibility.

Support is a given cost, determined by the level of support desired. It can be a block of hours for on-site support. (Note: If this is your choice, it is important to have a sign-in and sign-out sheet for both computer service personnel and your staff to sign and date each contact to accurately record the time used.) It can be a year-long contract for limited or unlimited phone support. Ideally, you will have support for both hardware and software from the same vendor, eliminating the possibility of each taking care of one part of the system while a problem remains unsolved. With support, have the vendor document in writing the maximum response time for your questions and problems. The documentation of the support hierarchy (the person you go to if your question is not answered or if you are unsatisfied with the support received after you have already paid for it) is essential.

Find out if the quoted price for the system is by the practice, the number of physicians, the total number of providers, or the number of user licenses. For instance, do you pay one price for the program for a software license for the entire practice, or do you have to buy a software license for each provider, thereby multiplying your cost by adding providers? Can you define the advance practice nurses who work in consultation with a physician as only needing one license? Often this is an overlooked, hidden cost.

How do you begin to choose a computer system?

In general, choices are an expression of views and values. When you get beyond that, it's brass tacks. The actual selection of a computer system is divided into four parts: preselection, software, hardware, and support (including implementation and training). Choose so that you are predisposed to find good in what you have chosen.

The First System Choice: Preselection

The preselection phase of choosing a computer system, i.e., making a rational, sound choice, begins with a narrow focus: Do you want a computer system? Like Pandora's box, this question opens many questions and information.

Your practice vision, mission statement, and business plan determine the goals you want to achieve. During this stage, keep an ongoing notebook dating, organizing, and classifying the information you acquire about information management. It is a good idea to talk your ideas through with coworkers and staff. They frequently agree with you, but it is your friends who are invaluable for they will argue. Establish a united approach with your office manager. Read as much as possible on the subject of current information management. Talk with peers who have similar practices. Ask questions in such a way that it is impossible to misunderstand the answers.

Interview past customers of the companies you consider buying from. Review current practice data to determine their transferability. Are the old and new programs written in the same language to make them compatible? Consider the ugly necessity of starting anew with updated reentered information (patient demographics, insurance company information, and provider data).

A good manager controls the implementation of directives. Assign an implementation leader from your staff for the start-up who will be training the computer person (or make that person the one who will maintain and upgrade the system).

Make a timeline for purchasing and implementing your computer. Include the installation and setup of software, the setup of hardware (to include necessary wiring), staff training, and the reestablishment of electronic data submission connections and credit card connections. The preselection phase combines information management needs with a budget for the system. Identify which information you want. Review information you have already gathered. Ask the staff for suggestions. Ask the vendor every question that enters your mind. Remember that the ultimate choice and responsibility are yours.

The Second System Choice:
The Selection of Computer Software

Software determines the minimal specifications required for hardware. Have your goals and budget firmly in mind. Read the information you choose to review: magazines, books, and the Internet. Gather the information together so that it can be easily and frequently referenced. When exhaustion takes over, ask your information management leader to continue, making sure he or she adheres to your timeline.

Review your priorities and the information you need to manage. Brainstorm with your staff. They have valuable input from a variety of astonishing perspectives. List how many people will be using the computer at one time. Establish a scale for comparing the important computer characteristics you are considering from the lowest (1 = worst, longest, slowest, etc.) to the highest (10 = best, shortest, fastest, etc.). Compare the capabilities of the systems. This is an excellent place to use an Excel-type table on your home computer to visualize comparisons. The difficult part is getting the right foot in the right stirrup to keep going forward. Comparisons help. They must include, but are not limited to, the following:

- Available applications (now and in the future)
- Ease of information input
- Ease of operation (ease of getting between necessary screens)
- Ease of training
- Availability of user help functions
  - ➤ Time required performing daily functions.
  - ➤ Required backup.
  - ➤ Level of confidentiality.
  - ➤ Method of upgrading.
  - ➤ Cost of an upgrade.
  - ➤ Data storage.
  - ➤ Internet use.
  - ➤ History of the company and software.
  - ➤ Logic and practicality of the screen layout.
  - ➤ Ease of changes made to the system (the way they are accomplished and the person who can make them).

> Description of which system parts are configured (screens, displays, reports, or content). If changes are made, does the vendor still support the system? Ease of audit trail for changes made to the system.
> Ease of setting system security.
> Ability to meet Health Information Portability and Accountability Act (HIPPA) regulations.
> Ease with which reports are generated.
> Number of reports that are generated at one time.
> Time required to generate and print monthly reports.
> Adequacy of reports producing the information needed to manage.
> The process of report creation when none exists.
> Possibility of accessing data from off-site workstations.
> Cost of each portion, possibility of electronic records, and prescription transmission.
> Ease of access to the database and possibility of interfacing with information management systems of local hospitals, laboratories, and x-ray facilities.

The Third System Choice: Computer Hardware and Support

The third choice is hardware. Review your vision, mission statement, business plan, and software requirements before talking the possibilities over with staff prior to the process of selecting hardware. For good hardware and support, present your options and ask what is feasible. Listen attentively and be alert to that one idea that will make a difference. Keep your goal tight and in sight as you establish a method of organizing the information gathered.

Ask your information management leader to join in the search for hardware and support. Then, after giving some thought to how well the shoe will bond with the sole, choose a hardware expert. This person will establish your minimum requirements: the processing power for the current and future workload, safety standards required in your environment, data storage capacity, the speed and capability of electronic data transmission for billing, and requirements for connectivity. In order to meet these goals, ask what additional equipment you can expect to connect to this system, such as a scanner, telephone answering system, the Internet, or a palm-computing device. In the process of obtaining two expert opinions about how to best meet your goal requirements, you will learn a lot. After the requirements have been determined, it's time to evaluate the actual hardware. Always ask for the opinions of peers and others in similar practices. Their mistakes become your experience.

Check your hardware warranty. What exactly (in writing and signed) does it cover? What is the usual life expectancy? What is the breakdown record? How are repairs made? Does the hardware need to be mailed to a central location, or is on-site service provided? Are loaners provided? What is their process for working with software vendors? Which software vendors are they used to working with? What is the capability for expansion? And last, but not least, what is the history of the company?

The Fourth System Choice: Implementation, Training, and Evaluation

In this final phase of computer selection, review your initial notes from the preselection phase, particularly those reflecting implementation, training, and evaluation. Evaluate the effectiveness of your information leader. Have your computer goals been met according to your timeline? You still have the opportunity to make changes where necessary, resetting timelines and objectives. At one moment, we may love our hair, our smile, our bloom—but we change for change is the key of our intelligence!

An effective information manager has a detailed, step-by-step implementation plan and timeline. To indicate agreement, the vendor needs to initial the implementation plan (including the timeline and cost). A written plan of improvement is a necessary part of the weekly progress meeting with your information leader. Arrange the computer implementation to minimally interrupt patient flow and employee function while keeping the cost of installation as low as possible. Competition in the computer field makes it possible to negotiate weekend installation at no additional charge.

It is safe to say the sun, moon, and trouble are all sure things. The prescient manager trains for trouble *and* success by explaining to the staff what is about to happen well in advance of disruptive computer installations and changes. The staff needs adequate preparation and time to feel the change to be prepared. Begin training the information leader upon the first contact with your selected vendor.

Prior to staff training, the information leader needs to set up the system. This includes the provider and insurance company profiles, charges, codes, visit types, reasons, and lengths. It also includes the patient recall system, collection system, and a schedule template for each provider (a skeleton plan for the schedule of visits, Monday through Friday—for example, beginning at 8 a.m. with 20-minute visits scheduled until noon, a respite until 2 p.m., followed by 30-minute visits scheduled until 5 p.m.). Be sure your information manager has transferred into the system all applicable patient data, including the individual existing patient appointments on the current provider schedule.

Staff training is best split in two halves. The first half describes and practices the necessary-to-operate functions. The second half of training follows a month later when you bring staff together to discuss any questions and problems they have identified. This is their opportunity to show interest and initiative. You have lived for this moment when your new system is in place.

Both you and your information leader know that implementation requires careful evaluation. Do the hard work of listening attentively. Establish an ongoing computer notebook, keeping track of the questions asked and answers given, the on-site and telephone support, and procedures and methods of operation, including dates and times. On preplanned periodic calendar dates, meet with your peers, information leader, office manager, staff, and daily staff information maintenance person. Your objective is to learn all you can about evaluating the computer system's adequacy, ease of operation, and future needs.

Information management in an advanced nursing practice is an ongoing challenge. It spurs your interest toward newer and more effective applications and hardware. You will discover yourself always pushing the system and staff toward your goal. Computers are no longer something we can do without. Ask questions until you are satisfied with the answers. Remember that the technology is there to assist you and improve the quality of the services you provide.

Quality Management 12

Cheryl W. Thompson

How is health care quality unique?

Patient health and satisfaction are the products of health care. They are difficult to measure. Although client outcomes are an essential indicator of quality, health care businesses rely on customer satisfaction. As you operate your practice in providing health care, you must understand and develop a quality measurement process that is consistent with your vision and leadership style. This chapter presents examples of various levels of quality management. The level you choose may depend on the requirements of regulatory agencies dealing with your practice. If your practice operates independent of certification by regulatory bodies, you are free to choose the level that is most manageable for you.

Is the provision of quality care inherent in the profession of nursing?

Yes! Most nurses are drawn to the profession because of their basic commitment to high-quality care. The ethical principles of professional practice imply a responsibility to provide care that is quality focused. These principles apply to any type of professional practice and include the following:

- **The principle of nonmaleficence.** Above all, do no harm.
- **The principle of beneficence.** Do good work.

The American Nurses Association (ANA) Code of Ethics for nurses is specific in declaring the nurse's responsibility to provide "quality health care."

What do all the quality terms mean?

Quality is defined as the "continuous striving for excellence." For a better understanding, it helps to review the history of quality in the health care industry. Monitoring with audits to assess quality originated in 1950. The following terms were used:

- **Quality assurance.**   A reactive process of evaluating care based on certain standards and implementing corrective measures
- **Quality indicator.**   Also referred to as a *benchmark* (a specific monitored incident or event)
- **Quality outcome.**   The specific goal of a quality process
- **Quality assessment.**   The process of measuring quality using the structure, process, and outcome focus
- **Quality improvement.**   The process of using quality measurements to identify problems and make changes

As the quality process in health care matured, a broader approach to quality was incorporated into the process; this involved all the previous processes in a comprehensive management pattern that revolved around a core commitment to providing the best and most cost-effective quality with continuous improvement throughout a health care practice. These terms, used synonymously, are as follows:

- Total quality
- Total quality management (TQM)
- Total quality improvement (TQI)
- Continuous quality improvement (CQI)

CQI is the term currently used in health care quality management. Achieving CQI is a huge endeavor. You may think, "I am not sure I am ready for that much work right now since I am just getting my business up and running." What is the minimum that must be done to meet quality requirements?

Basic quality for the APN practice is dictated by regulatory requirements. Established standards for licensure and certification are basic quality standards. These include requirements for maintaining the following:

- Current professional licensure
- Professional certification required by the state
- Certification by regulatory agencies such as the Clinical Laboratory Improvement Act (CLIA) for laboratory services and Medicare for provider status

You must determine which practice certifications are required. It is also helpful to know which other practices providing similar services incorporate quality control into their processes. This helps you stay competitive. APNs can easily meet the minimum requirements and be committed to providing quality service.

What is the next level?

Because the goal in health care is to provide the best and most cost-effective service to meet and exceed the expectations of the customer, gathering and acting on information about customer satisfaction is the next logical step for an APN.

To assess customer satisfaction, you first need to identify the customer. In a health care practice, the customer can fall under any of (or more than one of) the following categories.

Patients Who Are the Direct Recipients of Your Services

- Research shows that patients are more likely to choose a provider based on their own or an acquaintance's experience with a provider rather than data based on an agency's rating of the provider.
- Patient-satisfaction surveys, which are used to assess client satisfaction, are the most common method of data collection.
- Satisfaction information is gathered by attentive listening during APN-client interaction:

➤ Be attentive to comments made in passing about experiences with your practice.

➤ Communicate to your staff the need to listen attentively and to report on comments that clients make reflecting their impression of the practice's services.

Managed Care Organizations (MCOs) That Contract with You to Provide Services to Their Customers

- Your MCO contract defines the minimum quality you are expected to meet.
- Patient-satisfaction surveys are less helpful than alternative methods of data collection in assessing practice MCO customer satisfaction. You will need to
  ➤ Develop methods of communication with your MCO and request feedback from them, evaluating your services.
  ➤ Communicate to the practice staff their need to view the MCO as a customer.

Referral Sources

If all your patients are referred from one agency or organization, that referral source and the patient are your customers:

- Your referral source may define a minimum quality. However, in the next step, you will want to do more than the minimum requirement to maintain the referral source as a customer.
- Satisfaction surveys provide valuable information to your referral source. You need to use additional methods of assessing customer satisfaction such as the following:
  ➤ Maintain good communication between your practice and the referral source.
  ➤ Become involved in community projects that give you the opportunity to work professionally with your referral source.
  ➤ Communicate to your staff the need to view the referral source and patients as your customers.

What do you need to know about patient-satisfaction surveys?

Since surveys are difficult to write, in order to gather meaningful data, use a survey tool that has been developed and tested for its validity and reliability. Writing your own survey can introduce bias. Client-satisfaction surveys for acute care settings have been studied extensively. Find a tool that has been used for your setting. (See Appendix 3 for sample questions.)

Consider the following when evaluating a satisfaction survey:

- The reading level appropriate to your patient base
- Cultural relativity
- Language
- The ease of completion
- The ease of returning a completed survey

Typically, client-satisfaction surveys have a low return rate. Implement a system that will increase the likelihood that the survey will be completed and returned. Consider having the client complete the form before leaving the premises. Always provide return postage if surveys are mailed or taken home to be completed.

Then tabulate the results of returned surveys. APNs benefit by using a survey that has been developed and tested for its validity and reliability. Methods for data tabulation should be available with the survey.

The next step is to actually use the survey data. Patient-satisfaction surveys gathering dust on a desk serve little purpose in the quality process. Evaluate the current data and share it with your staff. It must be acted on for change to happen.

Make sure you give positive feedback to your staff from returned surveys. This improves staff job satisfaction, and, in turn, improves the quality of care your staff delivers. Be committed to doing everything possible in the interest of providing the highest quality patient care. What you give comes home to roost.

What quality process should you incorporate?

CQI is for you! CQI is the process of continual data collection, evaluation, and improvement. It is a philosophy, rather than a program, committed to the best practice at the lowest cost. CQI encourages input from a variety of sources before analyzing the input and determining ways to improve services based on the analysis. A CQI program focuses on prevention, problem solving, innovation, and creativity:

- A commitment to CQI is reflected throughout the practice and is evident in your vision and mission statements, organizational structure, job descriptions, and management style.
- CQI is a circular process:
  - ➤ Input is encouraged from patients, staff, referral sources, and the community.
  - ➤ Input is valued and critically evaluated by the entire practice.
  - ➤ All practice members work together systematically to develop plans to improve the care each member provides.
  - ➤ Evaluation is considered an input that flows back and around through the process.
- The comprehensive CQI program includes patients, staff, customers, services, and all aspects of care.
- A CQI program is proactive. Problems are identified before they occur.
- CQI occurs on a horizontal organization structure. Do not hinder staff input by reporting or using organizational mechanisms that create divisions.
- As a manager committed to CQI, APNs must
  - ➤ Manage using a democratic leadership style.
  - ➤ Continuously encourage and value input.
  - ➤ Commit to the administrative task of overseeing the process.

What are some components of CQI programs?

- Patient-satisfaction survey data that are carefully analyzed and incorporated in the review process.

- Recorded reviews of patient, financial, provider services, or administrative records include
  - ➤ A retrospective review to collect data.
  - ➤ A concurrent review to gather information relative to current practice standards.
  - ➤ A prospective of plans predicting future occurrences.
- Staff reviews committee that focuses on overall quality improvement. This committee could provide communication for input from your staff through various formats, such as formal regular work-hour meetings, informal lunch sessions, and a comment box with forms for input.
- Audits that focus on one specific aspect of care, such as contact pain assessment, risk assessment for specific illnesses, and preventive interventions at each contact.
- Risk management that focuses on problem prevention.
- Peer review.
  - ➤ Peer Review Organizations (PROs) are not yet as established for APN services as they have been for physician services.
  - ➤ Contract with a PRO in your area for quality review, or develop and conduct a constructive internal peer review.

How are patient records used in the CQI process?

The primary purpose of patient records is to document care and communicate patient information. Patient records are a key source of information in the CQI process. They are used to evaluate data, such as the following:

- The time spent with the patient
- The specific indicator being studied
- The evaluation of outcomes

Examine your APN philosophy and commitment to CQI before a record system is chosen and/or revised. This simplifies the retrospective review as well as data collection and analysis.

The patient record must allow for the easy extraction of data. Choose a record system that is developed and tested such as the OASIS or OMAHA systems. OASIS forms are available from the Centers for Medicare and Medicaid Services (CMS), formerly the Health Care Financing Administration (HCFA), Web site: www.cms.hhs.gov.

What is an example of a CQI model program?

A model program includes a structure, process, and outcome evaluation. Structure is the framework for your practice. Process evaluation is based on a review of systems that operate within the practice. The outcome evaluation identifies changes in patient status that occur as a result of the services provided. Outcome evaluation should receive the most attention in your CQI process. An outcome evaluation directs your review of structure and process as you work to improve outcomes.

Structure Evaluation

- **Policies and procedures.**   Are written policies and procedures accessible to all staff? Does a records review reflect that policies and procedures are followed?
- **Job descriptions.**   Are job descriptions clearly written? Do reviews reflect that job descriptions are followed? Do job descriptions reflect the CQI mission? In other words, is the communication of significant information to staff written in the job descriptions? Is there a job description that includes the responsibility of overseeing the CQI process?
- **Facilities.**   Are the facilities adequate for the services provided? Is there a welcoming and comfortable waiting area? Is the location accessible? Is there adequate space for record storage?
- **Supplies and equipment.**   Are the supplies needed for patient care easily accessible? Is the system for charging supplies set up so that supplies are charged accurately? Is equipment regularly cleaned, checked, and calibrated?

Process Evaluation

- **Peer review.**   This is done internally if more than one APN provides service in the practice. Develop a clear set of criteria for the
  review before beginning the peer review process. It is possible to
  contract for external peer review through a PRO; however, if the
  practice is unique, the PRO may not have standards that provide
  an appropriate review. A list of PROs in your area can be found
  at the American Health Quality Association (AHQA) Web site:
  www.ahqa.org.
- **Patient services.**   Ask the following questions: Does the scheduling system allow for an appropriate number of cancellations and
  emergency appointments each day? How long do patients wait to
  be seen? Are referrals to other providers made in a timely manner? Does the on-call answering service make appropriate decisions about when to call and when to hold messages?
- **CQI process.**   Is there a mechanism for input from your staff?
  Is there a mechanism for input from patients? When problems are
  identified, is there systematic planning, action, and evaluation?
- **Clinical practice.**   Clinical practice guidelines obtained from
  several sources such as AHRQ serve as a basis for the clinical
  practice evaluation. If an APN provides a unique service, it may
  be necessary to define clinical practice guidelines before conducting the evaluation.

Outcome Evaluation

- Outcome evaluation relies primarily on patient records and
  statistics.
- The desired outcome an APN chooses to measure depends upon
  the type of health care services offered. The effectiveness of an
  outcome evaluation depends on having a mechanism in your
  patient record system that clearly reflects the patient's status and
  the desired outcomes in a quantifiable form. Using a record system that reflects the patient's status at the time of the first assessment in a quantifiable way enhances the data collection for your
  outcome evaluation.

- Outcome evaluation should reflect the mission of your practice. For example, if your practice is a nurse-managed center with a mission to provide preventive health services, outcome measures are based on evaluating the occurrence of preventable illnesses.
- Outcome evaluation is set up to measure the frequency with which patients achieve established goals (outcomes). First, determine an acceptable level. For example, patients' records will reflect that short-term goals are met 90% of the time. If you collect data and find that short-term goals are met 50% of the time, begin the process and structure evaluation methods to gather more outcome information. What are the commonalities of patients when goals are not met? Do patients not return for service 50% of the time? Is the 50% nonreturn rate a problem? What measures can be taken to increase the return rate?
- Outcome evaluation implies that outcomes are directly related to the care provided. In fact, many other variables influence care. APNs need to be astute in defining outcome criteria evaluations that reflect the mission and goals of the practice.

How do you integrate CQI into the business plan you are writing?

- Vision and mission statements reflect a commitment to providing the highest quality at the lowest cost.
- Organizational structure incorporates the CQI vision and provides a good flow of useful information.
- Marketing plans reflect the following:
  - ➤ A commitment to providing the highest quality at the lowest cost
  - ➤ Clear patient identification
  - ➤ A description of a better and more cost-effective service than is currently provided by competitors
- Finance plans show the appropriate allocation of funds for implementing the CQI process.

You are operating an established practice.
How do you implement CQI?

- A strategic plan and/or annual review process provides the best opportunity to evaluate an APN's ability to incorporate CQI into the current organization.
- Evaluate the congruence of the mission statement with CQI.
- Describe the current quality process.

   ➤ Is it input driven or directed by regulatory requirements?
   ➤ Does the staff feel free to communicate concerns and make recommendations?
   ➤ Is the commitment to quality communicated to the staff?
- When implementing a systematic CQI process, focus on staff job satisfaction. Improving job satisfaction will improve care and quality. Begin by gathering information by asking the following questions:
   ➤ Does the staff feel valued?
   ➤ Can working conditions be improved?
   ➤ Does the staff have a place and time to communicate with each other and develop camaraderie?
   ➤ Do opportunities exist for professional development?
- Evaluate your own leadership style. Patriarchal, paternalistic, or autocratic leadership is incongruent with CQI.
- Focus on the processes of improved systems, communication, and patient care.
- Avoid being punitive when problems or shortcomings are identified.
- Begin practicing by using a philosophy that consistently values input in the direction of providing the best patient care.

Incorporating a CQI philosophy into the management of the APN practice with no time limit enables a vision to develop and be maintained. This is central to achieving continual improvement in developing a practice recognized for superior care.

Risk Management and Legal Issues

13

Susan Comstock

What must APNs consider in the legal aspects of a practice?

Starting any business can be fraught with legal perils. Service businesses, in particular, can be at additional risk because of problems arising not only from general business matters, but also from the unique relationship between clients and providers. The personality traits and qualities that make nurses successful in their chosen profession of caring are not necessarily the same personality traits and qualities that signify good business management. However, the basic knowledge and skills of running a business can be learned, and good consultants can provide the framework to avoid future problems and achieve success.

What type of attorney do you need?

The area of corporate practice consists of two basic attorney specialists: trial specialists and office specialists. When structuring a new business, an office specialist can help to prevent problems. Avoid using a friend or relative whose specialty is in another area of law, even if the hourly rate is lower. The experienced attorney spends fewer hours, and the overall cost will likely be lower.

How do you examine attorney credentials and make a decision?

One way to find a suitable attorney is to consult trusted friends and colleagues who have retained a business attorney. Ask for feedback.

Another way is to search a legal directory such as Martindale-Hubbell (available at your local library). Look for representative clients who provide the same type of professional health services you plan to provide. Ask the state bar association for a list of membership rosters of business law committees or a list of expert speakers on business start-ups. When you have a list from which to choose, look at the ranking of the law schools attended (reported annually in many places, including *U.S. News and World Report*). Arrange personal interviews with your candidates, ask what the fees are, request personal references, and determine how business services are arranged. Verify their relevant experience and the length of time they have practiced in this specific area. Ask for samples of work. Make sure the attorney has sufficient time and resources to provide services to you. The last decision is a gut decision: Do you trust this person for a long-term relationship? Do you have rapport? Does this person understand your goals? Once you have chosen an attorney, get a contract in writing, including the services, availability, projects, due dates, compensation, and whether or not you will be retaining the attorney after the initial services.

What are the implications and concerns affecting the legal structure?

When you start a business, you are setting up a separate legal entity, which will minimize your personal legal and financial liability. The ownership must be clear. This business entity must be structured in such a way that it can legally conduct the proposed business.

What are the four types of legal entities?

In *sole proprietorships*, the individual is the business and has no separate legal identity. The owner visits the county courthouse and files a *doing-business-as* (DBA) certificate. Business income taxes are filed on Schedule C on the owner's personal tax return. The owner is responsible for paying both the employer and employee half of social security taxes. Year-end losses are deducted from the owner's other taxable income. Quarterly estimated tax payments must be filed unless the owner or spouse has enough extra withheld at an employed job to cover the amount owed. More important, the owner's personal assets are unprotected legally as separate from the business.

Corporations are relatively easy to form and operate, but the owner may face double taxation both on corporate income and income earned as a shareholder. Double taxation is avoided by filing a *subchapter S corporation*, which is taxed similar to a partnership. Business liability is limited. However, an S corp has strict qualifying requirements. Professionals must often, by state law, form a specific type of corporation called a *professional corporation*. Decisions are made by officers, a board of directors, and stockholders (who, in some states, must be like-licensed professionals).

Partnerships involve a business relationship between two or more individuals or business entities. They are more difficult and costly to form. They do not shield owners from personal liability. Each partner is liable for the debts and legal liabilities of the other partners. Profits or losses are divided and applied to each partner's individual tax forms. Partnerships can create complex problems if one partner dies or wants to leave the partnership.

A *limited liability corporation* (LLC) is like a hybrid, blending the features of corporations and partnerships. It offers some liability exposure protection and can avoid paying federal income tax by using pass-through taxation. Professionals are eligible to form an LLC, but because it is a relatively new business form, not all states include it.

What state laws affect health professionals' corporate structuring?

Each state has special provisions that may affect the corporate structuring decisions by health professionals. Some state laws prohibit forming a professional corporation by professionals (such as nurses and physicians) with different forms of licenses. Some states ban the corporate practice of medicine and do not allow professional corporations. Most of these states will have some exceptions on this ban, such as free or nonprofit clinics or tax-exempt organizations operated as migrant or homeless health centers.

What special needs do you have in a health office lease agreement?

Standard forms fail to address the special leasing issues common in health care offices. These include the following:

- Use of hazardous materials and generation of biomedical waste
- Expense of building compliance with the Americans with Disabilities Act (ADA)
- Payment of landlord operating expenses when the tenant wants to provide their own janitorial and waste removal services
- Limitations of the landlord's rights to enter the premises to protect patient privacy
- Special building needs requiring specialized contractors with whom the landlord has no relationship and which would create a problem if the landlord wanted the tenant to later move to a different suite in the building

What are the important points of a collaborative practice agreement?

State law may require a collaborative practice agreement. APNs, physicians, or both may be legally responsible for drafting and filing the agreement. Review your state law about the APN scope of practice and prescriptive authority. Find out if the state board of nursing and/or board of medicine must approve the agreement. Some boards of nursing have sample agreements available. Discover if qualifications or limitations are placed on the collaborating physician. Some states limit the number of APNs a physician may supervise. Determine what services the APN will perform and in what setting they will be performed. Even if you know the collaborating physician, check references; ask about pending or past malpractice cases, the loss of hospital privileges, professional disciplinary actions, or the loss of Medicare participation.

Professional employment agreements: Employee or independent contractor?

If you need professional providers, you have the choice to hire them as employees or engage them as independent contractors. The primary element defining a worker as an independent contractor is the degree of oversight and control the employer has over the way the work is performed. The employer receives the following benefits from using individuals as independent contractors:

- Does not have to withhold income tax
- Does not have to pay social security tax
- Does not have to pay unemployment insurance tax
- Does not have to pay worker's compensation benefits
- Does not have to include employees in employer-sponsored benefit plans, including sick, holiday, and vacation pay
- Able to terminate the relationship for any reason specified in the agreement

However, independent contractor relationships can have serious legal and business issues, including federal regulations against fee splitting, fraud, and abuse. The employer has the following disadvantages from using individuals as independent contractors:

- The employer's malpractice insurance carrier may require the employer to include the contracting professional.
- Group pension plan issues may be affected.
- Medicare billing regulations generally prohibit a provider from billing Medicare for services performed by another provider.
- The employer may be subject to significant taxes and penalties if the IRS subsequently recharacterizes the relationship as employer-employee. The IRS uses 20 general factors to determine whether a professional is an employee or an independent

contractor, and is not bound by the definition in the employer contract.

Because of these and other complex issues, it is recommended that an attorney be consulted before hiring any professional as an independent contractor. The following are some factors to consider in a professional employment agreement:

- Do you want the position to be salaried, per hour, per day, or per patient as a percentage of either production or collections?
- What is the worth of services based on practice charges per patient visit and anticipated patient load?
- Is the employee expected to take call?
- What benefits, such as health insurance, vacation, sick leave, malpractice insurance, membership in a professional organization, journal subscriptions, and continuing education allowance and leave, are you willing to pay in addition to salary?
- Do you want to include a noncompete and antimoonlighting clause during the employment, and a noncompete clause after termination of the employment?
- What do you want to include for grounds for termination with cause or termination without cause by either party? Is a notice of intent to terminate required? Do you want to take into account possible future market conditions, mergers, consolidations, or dissolution? Will there be severance pay?
- In the event of a dispute, do you want the parties to go to binding arbitration?

It is worthwhile to have an attorney draw up a contract for the employment for all professionals in the practice. Make sure they have been thoroughly credentialed before they are hired.

Do you need a contract for nonprofessional employees?

Employment in most states is *at will*, which means the employee has a job at the will of the employer, and the employer may, at any time, fire the employee. The employee may also quit at any time. However, several recent court cases have begun eroding the at-will doctrine. Federal law provides protection to the employee against being fired on the basis of race, age, gender, or the exercise of free speech. A 3-month probationary period of employment is helpful. There are no protections for employers. If you want to ensure that an employee will stay for an established period of time, a contract is useful, specifying the conditions of employment, the duration of the contract, and provisions for a cause of discharge. An attorney can provide protection against a wrongful discharge action. A contract is considered automatically renewed if it does not specify that the terms revert to at will at the end of the identified period of employment or if the employee continues to provide the same services after the end of the contract.

Do you know the employment laws that apply to a practice?

ADA and Title VI of the Civil Rights Act

Employers with more than 15 employees are prohibited by Title 1 of the Americans with Disabilities Act of 1990 from discriminating against qualified individuals in hiring, firing, and other conditions of employment. A disabled person is defined as having a mental or physical impairment that substantially limits one or more major life activities. ADA also applies to hearing-impaired patients. Health care providers are required to provide and pay for auxiliary aids and services to ensure effective communication with patients who have disabilities affecting hearing, vision, or speech, so long as the cost does not impose undue hardship. Undue hardship is defined as an action that is excessively costly, extensive, substantial, or disruptive, or that would fundamentally alter the nature or operation of the business. An auxiliary aid or service, which exceeds the fee for treating the patient, is not by itself considered an undue hardship. Patients with limited English proficiency must be accommodated under Title VI of the Civil Rights Act. Written policies should exist on how to obtain interpreter services.

It is important to know how to write a fair job description, which will protect you from charges of discrimination in hiring or retaining a disabled worker. Identify the essential functions of each job. An essential function is a truly fundamental job duty. For example, a typist must be able to type, a receptionist must be able to deal with the public in person and on the telephone, and a phlebotomist must be able to draw blood. A function may also be essential if it is essential in your opinion. For instance, not all nurse practitioners may perform colposcopy or endometrial biopsy, but the APN may choose to identify it as an essential job function. It is important to identify minimum productivity standards, such as, in the case of the typist, the ability to type 60 words per minute. This helps prevent the APN from being forced to hire or continue employment for someone who is disabled and can now type only 3 words per minute.

The Fair Labor Standards Act (FLSA)

The FLSA exists to ensure fair compensation under the wage/hour law to employees. The FLSA requires employees be paid at least minimum wage for all hours worked and time and a half for all hours worked over 40 in a work week. An executive, administrative, or professional employee is classified as exempt from overtime requirements if paid on a predetermined salary basis, which is not subject to reduction due to variations in the quality or quantity of work performed. However, the employee does not need to be paid for a week in which the employee did no work. Overtime compensation may be paid to exempt employees without destroying their exempt status. If a worker files a complaint with the Department of Labor and an investigation by the Wage and Hour Division ensues, the employee is protected against retaliation.

Worker's Compensation

The worker's compensation system was established to provide an expeditious administrative program to provide benefits to an injured worker as a result of an industrial accident or occupational exposure. The benefits are to be awarded with minimum delay and regardless of fault. The system provides a direct remedy to the worker and limits litigation and exposure to the employer. Recovery for the injured employee is based upon a statutory scheme enacted by the legislature, which limits the employer's liability. The injured worker is limited to a percentage of his or her weekly earnings for temporary disability benefits and to a statutory schedule for permanent disability benefits. Under the worker's compensation system, the injured worker is not permitted to recover against the employer for negligence, pain and suffering awards, or punitive damages.

Drug Enforcement Administration (DEA) Regulations

The DEA is a federal agency whose mission is to enforce controlled substances laws and regulations and bring to justice anyone involved in the growth, manufacture, or distribution of controlled substances. You may obtain the *Mid-Level Practitioner's Manual: An Informational Outline of the Controlled Substances Act of 1970* from the DEA. It addresses registration requirements and guidelines for prescribers of controlled substances. There is also a listing of mid-level practitioner authorizations by state on the DEA Diversion Web site: www.deadiversion.usdoj.gov

Patient Confidentiality

Federal law requires health care providers to protect patient confidentiality. Special provisions are made for patients with mental health or substance abuse problems and nursing home residents. Patients should only be discussed in private areas, and their records should be kept out of view of other patients. Written documents should only be sent if the patient has signed a release form.

The Stark Acts

The Stark Acts prohibit physician referral of a patient covered by Medicare to designated health services when the physician or an immediate family member has a financial relationship with the facility providing those health services. There is an exemption that allows a physician to refer a patient to another physician in the same group practice without it being deemed a violation of the self-referral law. However, it is unclear whether this is intended to cover services by a nurse practitioner.

The Clinical Laboratories Improvement Act (CLIA)

CLIA has federal jurisdiction over clinical laboratories, including small office laboratories. Practices may file for a letter of exemption from CLIA if the laboratory tests performed are limited to fecal occult blood, urine pregnancy tests, blood glucose, urinalysis by dipstick, and office microscopy, such as wet mounts.

Occupational Safety and Health Administration (OSHA) and Health and Safety Management

Occupational safety and health may be administered by either a state agency or the federal OSHA agency. In addition, you will want to develop a health and safety policy and procedures manual for your practice that covers the following areas:

- Infection control
- Needle sticks and other sharps injuries
- The OSHA Bloodborne Pathogen Standard
- Occupational exposure to tuberculosis
- Occupational exposure to chemicals used in medical practice
- The OSHA Hazard Communication Standard
- Pharmaceuticals and controlled substances
- Medical gas handling and storage
- Medical equipment safety
- Servicing machines and equipment
- Personal protective equipment
- Latex glove allergy
- Hazardous and medical waste management
- Employee safety and health training
- Ergonomics
- Workplace violence
- Indoor air quality
- Patient safety program and emergency management
- Injury and illness reporting and investigating
- Worker's compensation and reporting requirements
- Program evaluation

Avoiding Medicare Billing Errors

The Department of Justice enforces the Center for Medicare and Medicaid Services (CMS) rules on billing for Medicare patients. The American Medical Association (AMA) jointly developed the office visit coding with CMS. If a visit has been up-coded from the appropriate coding and it is discovered through an audit, nurse practitioners can be charged with Medicare fraud and/or abuse. For specific questions on Medicare billing, download the Medicare Carriers Manual at www.cms.gov.

What specific issues of risk management, liability, and malpractice are of concern for practicing APNs?

Liability Risks in Writing Clinical Practice Guidelines

It is far better not to title documents that guide clinical practice as *protocols*, which defines specific steps in a particular procedure and has more medical-legal risk in court. Call them *guides to clinical practice*. Unfortunately, many state boards of nursing require that they be called *protocols*. If you practice in one of these states, work to change the language. The following elements should be included in these documents:

- Identification of all consulting physicians, backup physicians, and APNs in the practice
- Identification of all procedures beyond the core competencies and requirements to be met in order to practice them
- Identification of the scope of practice
- Definitions of independent and collaborative care, consultation, and referral
- Procedures for emergencies and the chain of command

The following elements should be left out of these documents:

- Standardized guidelines, unless you are sure they will be followed all of the time

- The words "never," "always," "will not," or "cannot"
- A laundry list of procedures and drugs
- Details that preclude clinical decision making in unexpected circumstances
- Safety issues or practices that could potentially limit a patient's availability to medical care

Special Concerns About Telephone Triage, Telehealth, and the Clinical Use of E-mail

Telephone triage

The goals of utilizing a telephone triage of patient concerns are to determine the severity of the problem, establish a working diagnosis, determine an intervention, and document the incident appropriately. It is paramount to determine how quickly the patient must be seen, where the patient should be seen, and who should see the patient. Standard litigation allegations include the failure to diagnose, improper or delayed treatment, and the failure to follow up. Additional malpractice allegations related to telephone triage include breaches of confidentiality, poor telephone procedures, and inadequate documentation. Problems in performing telephone triage include environmental distractions, cost concerns, and difficulty in establishing a reliable database due to the reduction of the communication process to only listening. In addition, past medical history from a chart and data from a physical examination or laboratory tests are not available. It is recommended that during office hours, only NPs or specifically trained RNs triage patient phone calls. After hours, the practitioner taking the call should have a copy of practice guidelines, drug reference guidelines, the phone numbers for the on-call collaborating physicians and hospital backup, 24-hour pharmacies, and hotlines and community resources. In addition, a clear communication method of ongoing patient issues to the succeeding on-call provider and a logistical mechanism for ensuring the timely placement of telephone triage notes into the patient chart must be in place.

Telehealth

According to the American Nurses Association (ANA), telehealth is the removal of time and distance barriers for the delivery of health care services or related health care activities. Some of the technologies used in telehealth include telephones, computers, interactive video transmissions, direct links to health care instruments, the transmission of images, and teleconferencing by telephone or video. Existing state laws regulating interstate practice of medicine or nursing have not kept pace with the growing use of telehealth by professionals and the increase in consumer health consultations via the Internet. However, nursing is far ahead of medicine in the recognition and amelioration of this problem. The National Council of State Boards of Nursing (NCSBN) adopted language for an Interstate Nurse Licensure Compact in 1998. This compact created a unified statement for nurses' licenses. Nurses will be able to practice telehealth in all states that adopt the compact. Currently, Arkansas, Maryland, and Utah have passed state laws allowing mutual recognition of out-of-state nursing licenses, and Nebraska, Texas, Wisconsin, and North Carolina have introduced similar legislation. Reimbursement for the practice of telehealth for Medicare recipients will be governed by rules proposed by the federal Department of Health and Human Services and CMS.

The clinical use of e-mail

The *Journal of the American Medical Informatics Association* has published guidelines on the clinical use of e-mail in connection with patients. Here is what they recommend:

- Establish the turn-around time for messages and do not use e-mail for urgent matters.
- Inform patients about privacy issues and include that message as part of the medical record.
- Establish the type of transactions (prescription refill, appointment scheduling, etc.) and the sensitivity of subject matter (HIV, mental health, etc.) permitted over e-mail.
- Request that patients put their name and patient identification number in the body of the message.
- Configure an automatic reply to acknowledge the receipt of messages.
- Print all messages with replies and the confirmation of receipt, and place them in the patient's paper chart.

- Send a new message to inform the patient that the request is complete.
- Maintain a mailing list of patients, but do not send group mailings where recipients are visible to each other. Use the blind copy software feature.

How do you deal with problem patients and patient complaints?

Many patient complaints have nothing to do with the care received, but are focused on front- or back-office issues. If it is difficult to make an appointment, waiting time is deemed excessive, prescription refill authorization takes days, billing mistakes are made, or telephone health inquiry responses are late (because medical records cannot be found), patients may be verbally unhappy or will simply vote with their feet and leave the practice. It is important to hire customer-oriented staff, have regular staff meetings about problem solving, and use patient-satisfaction survey tools proactively. In addition, an office manager or a staff person knowledgeable about customer service should be designated as the primary contact for unhappy patients and given the authority to exercise judgment in correcting a situation or offer appropriate tokens. For example, a teenager who comes in for a confidential pregnancy test and is dependent on an older friend for a ride may miss her ride because of unreasonable delays in the provision of services. This is an opportunity for the practice to offer a taxi pass for her transportation home.

The provider best deals with patient complaints about the clinical care received. Patients may not share the same set of beliefs the provider does about health and illness, and may not correctly interpret the quality of care given to them. In addition, a well-known subset of patients can become a challenge to risk management:

- Developmentally delayed patients should have a guardian present when counseling or teaching in order to avoid the risk of failure to obtain informed consent.
- Noncompliant patients should be questioned about why they have not followed recommendations, and their responses should be

documented in the chart as well as your attempts to increase compliance.

- Patients who are abusing substances and have conned their provider into prescribing the substance have sued the provider for contributing to their substance abuse.
- Polypharmacy patients who are on multiple medications should have been provided with a list of all medications, side effects, precautions, and dosing instructions reviewed at every visit. Make sure the patient is literate and has adequate eyesight. Consult with a pharmacist as needed.
- Patients with a generally positive review of systems should be evaluated for coping, dependency, and somatization issues. Prioritize addressing the complaints and repeat the review of system (ROS) at subsequent visits to see if complaints persist. Ensure that you follow the standard of care for each complaint.
- Medically high-risk patients with multisystem problems should be referred to a consultant as needed.
- Patients who discuss lawsuits against a previous provider are more likely to sue their current provider.

Do you need to provide patient chaperones?

The choice of whether or not to use a patient chaperone varies widely by community. Both same and opposite sex providers have been accused of improprieties. Particularly consider using a chaperone during physical examinations of unaccompanied minors. Sometimes the presence of a chaperone inhibits the free flow of information between patient and provider. Patient history questions are best asked when the chaperone is absent.

Do you need personal liability or personal injury insurance?

Personal liability insurance covers you for loss of property or injury to another as a result of your negligence. Check to see if you are covered for this under your homeowner or renter policy. Use professional malpractice insurance to cover nursing-related damages. Personal injury insurance, offered as an adjunct to some professional malpractice insurance policies, covers the following:

- False arrest, detention, or imprisonment
- Malicious prosecution
- Slander or libel
- Oral or written publication of material that violates a person's right to privacy
- Wrongful eviction from or entry into a privately occupied premise

How do you choose malpractice insurance?

Although traditionally APNs are less apt to be sued than their counterpart physicians, malpractice claims have been increasing. APNs are not immune to being named in a suit, even if they have not violated the standards of care and feel they have a good relationship with their patients. The determining factor in the decision to file a lawsuit is monetary—for instance, brain-damaged babies whose parents are without the financial resources to pay for lifelong care. Mandates in choosing a malpractice insurance carrier are as follows:

- Choose a financially strong company. Carriers can and do go bankrupt or out of business, sometimes in the middle of a trial. Make sure the company has at least a rating of A+ from Best's Guide to Insurance Companies.
- Choose an *occurrence policy*, if possible. This will cover you for claims filed in the future, even if your policy is no longer in force. A *claims-made policy* only covers you for claims made while the policy is in effect. You must continue coverage indefinitely by buying a tail even if you retire.
- Choose a policy, if possible, where legal costs are in addition to the limits of liability. Otherwise, if you have policy limits of $1,000,000 for a single claim and you have legal costs of $250,000, only $750,000 is paid on a $1,000,000 judgment against you, leaving you responsible for the remaining $250,000.

What is the National Practitioner Data Bank (NPDB)?

The NPDB is an information clearinghouse that collects and releases information related to professional competence and the conduct of physicians, dentists, and other health care practitioners. The NPDB was designed to restrict the ability of incompetent health care practitioners to move from state to state without disclosing previous incompetence. Access to information is granted to state licensing boards, hospitals, and other health care entities. Under certain circumstances, plaintiff attorneys may also obtain information. Medical malpractice insurers, defense attorneys, and the general public may not obtain the information. Individual practitioners may submit a Request for Information Disclosure form to find out whether they have been reported and what information is contained in the report. The following categories of information are collected:

- Medical malpractice payments
- Adverse licensure actions
- Adverse clinical privileges actions
- Adverse professional membership actions

What types of disciplinary action can a state board take?

A report of impairment, fraud, criminal activity, or gross negligence can be reported to a state board of nursing by a judge, patient, coworker, or supervisor. The state board will then send a letter to the APN stating that an investigation has been opened and a meeting must be arranged. After meeting with the APN, the investigator recommends to the board that the matter be dropped or an administrative hearing (which is similar to a trial) is necessary. The hearing officer then recommends to the board that the matter be dropped or the APN be disciplined. Discipline could include the revocation or suspension of one's license, or probation. Any investigation is an adversarial proceeding. An APN's right to due process requires attorney protection/representation throughout an investigation.

Ethical Issues Relative to an APN Practice

14

Ann Glasgow

Why should APNs be concerned with ethics?

With the emergence of the APN, a transformation occurred at the fundamental core of the educational process. The ability to process clinical information quickly and accurately became imperative for making decisions related to patient care and participating in a collaborative or independent practice. Sound clinical reasoning is the primary survival skill APNs must have to maintain themselves as effective providers of care.

APNs are responsible, legally and ethically, for the quality of care provided to a patient. Accountability is implied in the complete obligation to the patient and in the relationship between the patient and the nurse. The main concern inherent in this relationship is the care of the whole patient (including humanistic, moral, and ethical values), which reaches beyond the patient relationship to include family, community, legal authorities, and professional colleagues.

Professional accountability is merged with the continuum of greater nursing complexity in the health care environment, which extends beyond the traditional moral or ethical and medical models to include concepts of duty, autonomy, service, competence, authority, and commitment. The greatest impacts on these concepts come from barriers imposed by unconstructive collaborative relationships between APNs and physicians and by constraints imposed by the health care system.

The current trends toward APNs are responsive to the market's expansion to cover the needs for health care and other systems delivering services. Accountability is measured against established standards for education and expertise. The parameters of accountability and authority for the APN are clearly defined within the profession's standards and scope of practice, which are regulated at the state level. Truly accountable practices are shaped by values of compassion significant to the nurse-patient relationship and excellence in skills, ethical obligations, and professional standards. Ethical principles are found at the nucleus of accountability in an APN practice.

What ethical principles are pertinent to an APN practice?

The conceptual framework and moral dimension of accountability for an APN practice are based on certain ethical principles integral to education and practice. Traditional principles such as nonmaleficence, beneficence, autonomy, justice, and veracity can be expanded to include concepts such as advocacy, fidelity, care, compassion, and human dignity. For an understanding of pertinent philosophic concepts relative to ethical practices, these key principles are defined as follows:

- **Autonomy.** The right to make one's own decisions
- **Justice.** Applying fairness to everyone, sound reason, and rightfulness of decisions and actions
- **Rights.** The belief that everyone has certain inalienable rights simply by being human
- **Formalism.** The strict adherence to customs such as religious tenets; no swaying from the straight and narrow path
- **Beneficence.** The duty to do good and not harm others
- **Nonmaleficence.** The duty to do no harm to others
- **Freedom.** Refers to the belief that everyone is entitled to make choices and holds that each person is responsible for the consequences of his or her actions
- **Fidelity.** The duty to be true and loyal to others
- **Veracity.** The act of telling the truth
- **Advocacy.** The act of pleading one cause for another
- **Privacy.** Privacy belongs to each person and cannot be taken away from that person unless he or she wants it
- **Confidentiality.** The idea that the information shared with other persons will not be spread abroad and will be used only for the purposes intended

What is the purpose of the Nursing Code of Ethics?

Ethics refers to the practices, beliefs, and standards of behavior of a certain group. These standards are described in the group's code of professional conduct. The Nursing Code of Ethics developed by the American Nurses Association (ANA) sets forth a set of ethical principles that reflect moral judgments over time and serve as a standard for their professional actions, which are usually higher than legal standards. The Nursing Code of Ethics has the following purposes:

- To inform the public about the minimum standards of the profession and to help the public understand professional nursing conduct
- To provide a sign of the profession's commitment to the public it serves
- To outline the major ethical considerations of the profession
- To provide general guidelines for professional behavior
- To guide the profession in self-regulation
- To remind nurses of the special responsibility they assume when caring for patients

Inherent to ethical dilemmas are the frequent conflicts between the rights and responsibilities involving human rights issues. The commitment to provide services with respect to human dignity (as stipulated in the Code for Nurses with Interpretive Statements) is based on respect for human beings as an end in itself and as a holder of freedoms, claims, and entitlements. Translating this view of human beings into specific nursing action involves the process of reasoning about what ought to be done for the patient, and is accompanied by observations and judgments about patient response and technical expertise in the actual delivery of care as a necessary component of nursing practice (ANA, 2002). The following beliefs, which help define human rights, shape the activities for the ANA Center for Ethics and Human Rights (CEHR):

- Human beings, as ends in themselves, deserve respect and therefore deserve nursing services that are equitable in terms of accessibility, availability, affordability, and quality.
- Justice requires that the differences among persons and groups be valued. When those differences contribute to the unequal distrib-

ution of the quality of nursing and health care, remedial action is obligated.

- The principle of justice applies to nurses as both providers and recipients of care. The ANA is committed to addressing the need for racial and ethnic diversity among nurses. Such diversity is a critical element in providing fair and equitable care.
- Because nursing care is an essential but sometimes limited commodity, the allocation of care is a pressing issue that is not effectively addressed when specific individuals are excluded or when the burdens of limited access are borne by particular groups.

The APN has at least three responsibilities:

- The careful delivery of nursing care in a way that meets the needs of the individual and is consistent with the goals of the individual in respect to the level of health and quality of life
- Social action and reform to increase the availability of nursing care and to facilitate access to needed health care for all
- Patient education and advocacy to ensure that individuals are aware of all options and their consequences and can make informed choices about their health care

In addition, APNs must advance and protect their own human rights, including the right to be fairly compensated for the services rendered, the right to control the quality of practice, the right to engage in whistle-blowing when necessary without reprisal, and the right to engage in an independent practice.

What defines an ethical dilemma?

Ethical problems are created as a result of changes in society, advances in technology, conflicts within roles, and conflicts with loyalties and obligations to patients, families, employees, physicians, and other nurses. When making ethical decisions, an APN should consider the Nursing Code of Ethics together with the more unified ethical theory, ethical principles, and relevant data about each situation. An ethical dilemma is the choice between two or more equally justifiable alternatives. These dilemmas are identified by the types of ethical problems encountered as either decision-focused problems or action-focused problems. Decision-focused problems focus on "What should I do?" whereas action-focused problems ask "What can I do?" or "What risks am I willing to take to do what is right?"

Why should APNs use a decision-making model?

Decision-making models, serving as guidelines in resolving an ethical dilemma, include

- Facts of the specific situation
- Ethical theories and principles
- The Nursing Code of Ethics
- Patient rights
- Personal values
- Factors that contribute to, or hinder one's ability, to make or enact a choice, such as cultural values, societal expectations, the degree of commitment, the lack of time, the lack of experience, ignorance or fear of the law, and conflicting loyalties

An important first step in ethical decision making is to ensure the problem has ethical or moral content. The following criteria are used to determine whether a moral situation exists:

- There is a need to choose between alternative actions that conflict with human wants and necessities and the welfare of others.
- The choice to be made is guided by universal moral principles or theories, which can provide justification for the action.
- A process of weighing reason guides the choice.
- The decision must be freely and consciously chosen.
- The choice is affected by personal feelings and by the particular context of each situation.

The most important decision is determining who should make the decision. When the decision maker is the patient, the nurse functions in a supportive role. Patients need knowledge about the consequences attending various courses of action. The following questions are helpful to determine the ownership of a problem:

- For whom is the decision being made?
- Who should be involved in making the decision and why?
- What criteria (social, economic, psychological, physiological, or legal) are used to decide who makes the decision?
- What degree of consent does the subject need?

Although pertinent ethical obligations are prevalent between the APN and the patient, other factors between an employer and collaborative physician must also be taken into account in the decision-making process. The following actions serve as guidelines in this process:

1. Collect facts relevant to the situation.
2. Analyze the facts and determine who is involved in making the decision.
3. Clarify issues using associated ethical principles, theories, laws, and policies.
4. Interpret the information into a concise situation statement.
5. Develop a list of actions with associated projected outcomes for everyone involved with the situation.
6. For each action and outcome, analyze the advantages and disadvantages.
7. Strategically identify a plan for the action selected.
8. Make a decision.
9. Implement the plan.
10. Evaluate the results to determine if the selected plan is successful. If the outcome is not what is wanted, look at other options and adapt to achieve a better outcome.

What strategies enhance the ethical decision-making process?

In all situations, APNs are ethically obligated to maintain a nonjudgmental attitude, be honest, and protect the patient. To enhance ethical decision making, the following strategies are pertinent:

- Become aware of your own values and the ethical aspects of nursing situations.
- Find an appropriate decision-making process to use in daily nursing situations.
- Be familiar with the Nursing Code of Ethics, patient rights, and scope of practice.
- Understand the values of patients and health care professionals.
- Participate on ethics committees and peer review committees.
- Be familiar with specific ethical issues currently undergoing scrutiny.

When are APNs ethically obligated to provide care?

APNs in an independent practice who enter into contracts for service with patients are in a binding contract once treatment begins. First, a contract is an exchange of promises between two people who are legally capable of making a binding agreement. Second, to be valid, a contract must offer something and contain an acceptance of that offer. A third requirement is consideration: Something of value must be exchanged between the parties. State and federal statutes prohibit discrimination on the basis of gender, age, race, nationality, religion, marital status, or certain health conditions. In some legal cases, people with HIV or AIDS have won monetary settlements from health care providers. Cases range from the outright refusal to treat patients to the refusal to treat in the provider's office with an offer to treat the patient in a hospital or other facility.

The ANA Committee on Ethics establishes that when a person meets the following four criteria, a nurse is obligated to provide care:

- The patient is at significant risk of harm, loss, or damage if the nurse does not assist.
- The nurse's intervention or care is directly relevant to preventing harm.
- The nurse's care will probably prevent harm, loss, or damage to the patient.
- The benefits the patient will gain outweigh any harm the APN might cause, providing care does not present more than a minimal risk to the nurse.

If the patient is purposefully uncooperative, the APN has the right to refuse treatment and refer the patient to a physician or specialist for the specific problems identified by the patient. In this way, another opinion is obtained or an observation is uncovered that may have been missed in the APN's encounter with the patient. So often "red herrings" get in the way of patient communication.

Why should APNs be concerned about applied ethical issues?

With the emergence of the APN, a definite change in the scope of practice has led to a direct involvement with central ethical issues requiring complex ethical decisions. With the public's alertness to key issues, it is important that the APN is knowledgeable about the current ethical outcomes of dealing with patients, family, and colleagues confronted with related ethical dilemmas.

In general, human rights are justified claims by individuals and groups on individuals or society. According to ANA guidelines,

- **Liberty rights.** The responsible exercise of freedom exemplified in the Bill of Rights and the U.S. Constitution and the first-generation rights
- **Claim rights.** Assertions that call for a fair share of resources, services, and assistance of others in the realization of human potential and in protection from harm and the second-generation rights subject to legislation

When care provided by APNs is viewed as a resource, it must be distributed fairly and equitably to meet the needs of a population group. Achieving fairness and equity in the distribution of services is a continuous challenge for the professional association and one that often requires APNs to act as advocates for their patients.

In addition, APNs engage in a variety of activities that have the potential of impinging on the rights of other human beings, such as in organized research using animal or human subjects. Increasingly, the borderline between usual and expected and experimental clinical practices is becoming blurred. As the scope of nursing practice increases in complexity, nursing as a profession realizes the importance of concerning itself with the human rights of all persons who receive services including those who are participants in clinical research.

Professional nurses should support the patient's right to self-determination. Ideally, the patient should make the decision about advance (end-of-life) directives with the family and the primary provider prior to admission to a hospital. The formation of advance directives is an important decision and inevitably involves nurses who are the most omnipresent professionals in health care facilities. It is imperative that nurses facilitate the patient's (and family's) decision-making process about end-of-life care. An APN is one of several health care professionals with a responsibility to ensure that advance care directives initiated by the patient are current and reflect the patient's choices. The process of facilitating patient self-determination regarding end-of-life decisions includes the ability to evaluate changes in the patient's perspective and state of health. The nurse has a responsibility to facilitate informed decision making including, but not limited to, advance directives.

The ANA (2002) recommends that the APN advance directive assessment include the following questions:

- Do you have basic information about advance care directives, including living wills and durable power of attorney?
- Do you want to initiate an advance care directive?
- If you have already prepared an advance care directive, can you provide it now?
- Have you discussed your end-of-life choices with your family and/or designated surrogate and health care team worker?

The role of the APN is critical to implementing the Patient Self-Determination Act. Each nurse should know the laws of the state in which he or she practices, pertaining to advance directives, and should be familiar with the strengths and limitations of the various forms of advance directives.

What current medical ethics issues affect APN practices for this century?

Key contentious areas confronting APNs are the issues of rights and needs of the patient and protection of patients from harm. The following are examples of ethical dilemmas:

- **Mortality.** This refers to the determination of the quality of life and when life has ended. The key definition adopted by the United States in 1981 speaks to the irreversible cessation of circulatory and respiratory functions and irreversible cessation of all functions of the entire brain. The question of mortality points to cases such as the Quinlan case and those judicially questioned in the Kevorkian cases of assisted suicide.
- **Reproductive medicine.** This refers to the determination of birth-control issues (such as abortion) and infertility measures (such as in vitro fertilization). Laws that determine the rights of the mother and the time period in which an abortion can be performed are abortion issues.
- **Genetic technology issues.** These involve the determination of what human manipulative procedures are legally permissible in society. The greatest concern has been mapping the human genome, which could lead to human cloning.
- **Provider-patient issues.** These involve key issues that place the provider at risk when treating the patient. Scrutinize, evaluate, and adhere to the state laws concerning the patient's right to refuse treatment. As AIDS cases increase, many providers, in an effort to avoid treating these cases, directly deny care and therefore discriminate against persons suffering with this disease.
- **Human experimentation.** The key issue is the monitoring of clinical trials and experiments involving humans. Internal Review Board (IRB) approval is required prior to any such experiment enabling the agency to determine if the patient might be put at risk of harm.
- **Organ and tissue transplants.** Over recent years, significant issues have been raised about the practice of transplantation. Success, which brings new life and hope to patients who would have

died if these procedures had not been available, carries with it a measure of acceptance by society. Ethical uncertainty continues to evolve around human embryonic stem cells using human embryos. This is traceable to key abortion issues. Is it morally acceptable to extinguish the life of a living human and use those cells to give life to another human?

With the emergence of the 21st century, issues continue to be unresolved. As the aging population grows, the costs and life-sustainable measures of the health care system are affected proportionately, requiring debate and choices. The practicing APN needs to be secure in his or her personal values and thoughts about key ethical dilemmas while keeping abreast of public debates and changes in the law. An ethical decision-making APN worksheet helps address the issue of logical choice. (See Appendix 6 for the ethical decision-making APN worksheet.)

Where can APNs find additional ethical resources and references?

A wealth of information for APNs is available on the Internet. Visit the following Web sites:

ANA	www.ana.org
American Medical Association (AMA)	www.ama.org
International Council of Nurses	www.icn.org
Online Journal of Issues in Nursing	www.nursingworld.org/ojin/ethical/ethics
The Internet Journal of Advanced Nursing Practice	www.icaap.org/luicode?99.1.2.4
	www.acponline.org
	www.aslme.org
	www.cwru.edu/med/bioethics
	www.ethics.ube.ca/resources
	www.jcaho.org
	www.nih.gov.ethical

Certifying Boards for Specific Practice Areas

- **American Academy of Nurse Practitioners (AANP)**
  Certification Program
  Capitol Station, P.O. Box 12926
  Austin, TX 78711
  Phone: (512) 442-4262 ext. 214
  Fax: (512) 442-5221
  Web site: www.AANP.org or www.ana.org/aanp

  For the Adult Nurse Practitioner (ANP) and Family Nurse Practitioner (FNP)

- **American Nurses Credentialing Center (ANCC)**
  600 Maryland Avenue, SW, Suite 100 West
  Washington, DC 20024-2571
  Phone: (800) 284-2378
  E-mail: ANCC@ana.org—Please do not use e-mail address to request a
  catalog.

  For the Acute Care Nurse Practitioner (ACNP), ANP, FNP, General Nurse
  Practitioner (GNP), Psychiatric Clinical Nurse Practitioner (PsychCNS), and
  Pediatric Nurse Practitioner (PNP)

- **National Certification Board of Pediatric Nurse Practitioners**
  and Nurses (NCBPNP/N)
  800 South Frederick Avenue, Suite 104
  Gaithersburg, MD 20877-4150
  Phone: (301) 330-2921 and (888) 641-2767
  Fax: (301) 330-1504
  For the PNP

- **National Certification Corporation for the Obstetric, Gynecologic, and**
  Neonatal Nursing Specialties (NCC)
  645 North Michigan Avenue Suite 1058
  Chicago, IL 60611
  Phone: (800) 367-5613 or (312) 951-0207

  For the Neonatal Nurse Practitioner (NNP) and Women's Health Care Nurse
  Practitioner (WHCNP)

State Licensing Agencies

Alabama Board of Nursing
P.O. Box 303900
770 Washington Avenue, RSA Plaza,
Suite 250
Montgomery, AL 36130
Phone: (334) 242-4060
Fax: (334) 242-4360
Web site: www.abn.state.al.us

Alaska Board of Nursing
Department of Community and
Economic Development
Division of Occupational Licensing
3601 C Street, Suite 722
Anchorage, AK 99503
Phone: (907) 269-8161
Fax: (907) 269-8156
Web site: www.dced.state.ak.us

Arizona State Board of Nursing
1651 E. Morten Avenue, Suite 150
Phoenix, AZ 85020
Phone: (602) 255-5092
Fax: (602) 255-5130
Web site: www.azboardofnursing.org

Arkansas State Board of Nursing
University Tower Building
1123 S. University, Suite 800
Little Rock, AR 72204
Phone: (501) 686-2700
Fax: (501) 686-2714
Web site: www.state.ar.us

California Board of Registered Nursing
P.O. Box 944210
Sacramento, CA 94244
Phone: (916) 322-3350
Fax: (916) 327-4402
Web site: www.rn.ca.gov

Colorado Board of Nursing
1560 Broadway, Suite 670
Denver, CO 80202
Phone: (303) 894-2430
Fax: (303) 894-2821
Web site: www.dora.state.co.us

Connecticut Board of Examiners for Nursing
Division of Health Systems Regulation
410 Capitol Avenue, MS# 12HSR
P.O. Box 340308
Hartford, CT 06134
Phone: (860) 509-7624
Fax: (860) 509-7286
Web site: www.state.ct.us/dph

Delaware Board of Nursing
861 Silver Lake Boulevard
Cannon Building, Suite 203
Dover, DE 19903
P.O. Box 1401
Phone: (302) 739-4522
Fax: (302) 739-2711
Web site:
www.professionallicensing.state.de.us

District of Columbia Board of Nursing
825 N. Capital St. NE
Washington, DC 20001
Phone: (202) 442-4776
Fax: (202) 442-9431
Web site: www.dchealth.de.gov

Florida Board of Nursing
4052 Bald Cypress Way
Tallahassee, FL
Phone: (850) 245-4125
Fax: (850) 245-4172
Web site: www.doh.state.fl.us

Georgia Board of Nursing
166 Pryor Street, S.W.
Atlanta, GA 30303
Phone: (404) 656-3943
Fax: (404) 657-7489
Web site: www.sos.state.ga.us

Guam Board of Nurse Examiners
P.O. Box 2816
Agana, GU 96910
Phone: (671) 475-0251
Fax: (671) 477-4733

Hawaii Board of Nursing
Professional and Vocational Licensing
Division
P.O. Box 3469
Honolulu, HI 96801
Phone: (808) 586-2695
Fax: (808) 586-2689
Web site: www.state.hi.us

Idaho Board of Nursing
280 N. 8th Street, Suite 210
P.O. Box 83720
Boise, ID 83720
Phone: (208) 334-3110
Fax: (208) 334-3262
Web site: www.state.id.us

Illinois Department of Professional
Regulation
James R. Thompson Center
100 West Randolph, Suite 9-300
Chicago, IL 60601
Phone: (312) 814-2715
Fax: (312) 814-3145
Web site: www.dpr.state.il.us

Indiana State Board of Nursing
Health Professions Bureau
402 W. Washington Street, Room W041
Indianapolis, IN 46204
Phone: (317) 232-2960
Fax: (317) 233-4236
Web site: www.state.in.us/hpb

Iowa Board of Nursing
State Capitol Complex
1223 East Court Avenue
Des Moines, IA 50319
Phone: (515) 281-3255
Fax: (515) 281-4825
Web site:
www.state.ia.us/government/nursing

Kansas State Board of Nursing
Landon State Office Building
900 S.W. Jackson, Suite 551-S
Topeka, KS 66612
Phone: (913) 296-4929
Fax: (913) 296-3929
Web site: www.ksbn.org

Kentucky Board of Nursing
312 Whittington Parkway, Suite 300
Louisville, KY 40222
Phone: (502) 329-7006
Fax: (502) 329-7011
Web site: www.kbn.state.ky.us

Louisiana State Board of Nursing
3510 N. Causeway Boulevard, Suite 501
Metairie, LA 70002
Phone: (504) 838-5332
Fax: (504) 838-5349
Web site: www.lsbn.state.la.us

Maine State Board of Nursing
158 State House Station
Augusta, ME 04333
Phone: (207) 287-1133
Fax: (207) 287-1149
Web site: www.state.me.us/nursingbd

Maryland Board of Nursing
4140 Patterson Avenue
Baltimore, MD 21215
Phone: (410) 764-5124
Fax: (410) 358-3530
Web site: www.mbon.org

Massachusetts Board of Registration in Nursing
239 Causeway St., Suite 500
Boston, MA 02114
Phone: (617) 727-9961
Fax: (617) 727-2197
Web site: www.state.ma.us

State of Michigan CIS/Office of Health Services
Ottawa Towers North
611 W. Ottawa, 4th Floor
Lansing, MI 48933
Phone: (517) 373-9102
Fax: (517) 373-2179
Web site: www.cis.state.mi.us

Minnesota Board of Nursing
2829 University Avenue SE, Suite 500
Minneapolis, MN 55414
Phone: (612) 617-2270
Fax: (612) 617-2190
Web site: www.nursingboard.state.mn.us

Mississippi Board of Nursing
1935 Lakeland Dr., Suite B
Jackson, MS 39201
Phone: (601) 987-4188
Fax: (601) 364-2352
Web site: www.msbn.state.ms.us

Missouri State Board of Nursing
3605 Missouri Boulevard
P.O. Box 656
Jefferson City, MO 65102
Phone: (573) 751-0681
Fax: (573) 751-0075
Web site: www.ecodev.state.mo.us

Montana State Board of Nursing
Arcade Building, Suite 4C
111 North Jackson
Helena, MT 59620
Phone: (406) 444-2071
Fax: (406) 444-7759
Web site: www.com.state.mt.us

Department of Health and Human Services Regulation and Licensure Credentialing Division— Nursing/Nursing Support Section
301 Centennial Mall South
P.O. Box 94986
Lincoln, NE 68509
Phone: (402) 471-4376
Fax: (402) 471-3577
Web site: www.hhs.state.ne.us

Nevada State Board of Nursing
1755 East Plumb Lane, Suite 260
Reno, NV 89502
Phone: (702) 786-2778
Fax: (702) 322-6993
Web site: www.nursingboard.state.nv.us

New Hampshire Board of Nursing
78 Regional Drive, Building B
Concord, NH 03301
Phone: (603) 271-6599
Web site: www.state.nh.us

New Jersey Board of Nursing
124 Halsey Street, 6th Floor
P.O. Box 45010
Newark, NJ 07101
Phone: (201) 504-6586
Fax: (201) 648-3481
Web site: www.state.nj.us

New Mexico Board of Nursing
4206 Louisiana Boulevard, NE, Suite A
Albuquerque, NM 87109
Phone: (505) 841-8340
Fax: (505) 841-8347
Web site: www.state.nm.us

New York State Board of Nursing
State Education Building, 2nd Floor
Albany, NY 12234
Phone: (518) 474-3817
Fax: (518) 474-1449
Web site: www.nysed.gov

North Carolina Board of Nursing
3724 National Drive
Raleigh, NC 27602
Phone: (919) 782-3211
Fax: (919) 781-9461
Web site: www.ncbon.com

North Dakota Board of Nursing
919 South 7th Street, Suite 504
Bismarck, ND 58504
Phone: (701) 328-9777
Fax: (701) 328-9785
Web site: www.ndbon.org

Ohio Board of Nursing
17 South High Street, Suite 400
Columbus, OH 43215
Phone: (614) 466-3947
Fax: (614) 466-0388
Web site: www.state.oh.us

Oklahoma Board of Nursing
2915 N. Classen Boulevard, Suite 524
Oklahoma City, OK 73106
Phone: (405) 525-2076
Fax: (405) 521-6089
Web site: www.youroklahoma.com

Oregon State Board of Nursing
800 NE Oregon Street,
Box 25, Suite 465
Portland, OR 97232
Phone: (503) 731-4745
Fax: (503) 731-4755
Web site: www.osbn.state.or.us

Pennsylvania State Board of Nursing
124 Pine Street
P.O. Box 2649
Harrisburg, PA 17105
Phone: (717) 783-7142
Fax: (717) 783-0822
Web site: www.dos.state.pa.us

Commonwealth of Puerto Rico
Board of Nurse Examiners
800 Roberto H. Todd Avenue, Room
202, Stop 18
Santurce, PR 00908
Phone: (787) 725-7506
Fax: (787) 725-7903

Rhode Island Board of Nursing
Registration and Nursing Education
Cannon Health Building
Three Capitol Hill, Room 104
Providence, RI 02908
Phone: (401) 277-2827
Fax: (401) 277-1272
Web site: www.health.state.ri.us

South Carolina State Board of Nursing
110 Centerview Drive, Suite 202
Columbia, SC 29210
Phone: (803) 896-4550
Fax: (803) 896-4525
Web site: www.llr.state.sc.us

South Dakota Board of Nursing
3307 South Louise Avenue
Sioux Falls, SD 57106
Phone: (605) 362-2760
Fax: (605) 362-2768
Web site: www.state.sd.us

Tennessee State Board of Nursing
426 Fifth Avenue North
Cordell Hull Building, 1st Floor
Nashville, TN 37247
Phone: (615) 532-5166
Fax: (615) 741-7899
Web site: http://170.142.76.180/
bmf-bin/BMFproflist.pl

Texas Board of Nurse Examiners
333 Guadalupe #3-460
Austin, TX 78701
Phone: (512) 305-6843
Fax: (512) 305-7401
Web site: www.bne.state.tx.us

Utah State Board of Nursing
Division of Occupational and
Professional Licensing
Heber M. Wells Building, 4th Floor
160 East 300 South
Salt Lake City, UT 84111
Phone: (801) 530-6628
Fax: (801) 530-6511
Web site: www.commerce.state.ut.us

Vermont State Board of Nursing
109 State Street
Montpelier, VT 05609
Phone: (802) 828-2396
Fax: (802) 828-2484
Web site: http://vtprofessionals.org

Virgin Islands Board of Nurse Licensure
Veterans Drive Station
St. Thomas, VI 00803
Phone: (340) 776-7397
Fax: (340) 777-4003

Virginia Board of Nursing
6606 W. Broad Street, 4th Floor
Richmond, VA 23230
Phone: (804) 662-9909
Fax: (804) 662-9943
Web site: www.dhp.state.va.us

Washington State Nursing Care Quality Assurance Commission
Department of Health
1300 Quince Street SE
Olympia, WA 98504
Phone: (360) 753-2686
Fax: (360) 586-2165
Web site: www.doh.wa.gov

West Virginia Board of Examiners for Registered Professional Nurses
101 Dee Drive
Charleston, WV 25311
Phone: (304) 558-3596
Fax: (304) 558-3666
Web site: www.state.wv.us

Wisconsin Department of Regulation and Licensing
1400 E. Washington Avenue
P.O. Box 8935
Madison, WI 53708
Phone: (608) 266-2112
Fax: (608) 267-0644
Web site: www.drl.state.wi.us

Wyoming State Board of Nursing
2020 Carey Avenue, Suite 110
Cheyenne, WY 82002
Phone: (307) 777-7601
Fax: (307) 777-3519
Web site: http://nursing.state.wy.us

Patient Survey of Health Care for a Practice

Circle one of the following choices:

1. Overall, how would you rate the medical clinic visit?
   Excellent   Fair
   Very good   Poor
   Good

2. Would you please explain why you rated it fair/poor?
   Provider didn't listen to patient/family
   Long wait
   Unfriendly/uncaring staff
   Given wrong medication
   Misdiagnosed

3. How would you rate your satisfaction as you made an appointment for the visit?
   Excellent   Fair
   Very good   Poor
   Good

4. How would you rate your satisfaction with the reception you/your family member received at this clinic?
   Excellent   Fair
   Very good   Poor
   Good

5. If you were seen by an Advanced Practice Nurse (APN), how would you rate the overall quality of care provided?
   Excellent   Fair
   Very good   Poor
   Good   Did not see APN

6. If you were seen by a physician, how would you rate the overall quality of care provided?

Excellent	Fair
Very good	Poor
Good	Did not see physician

7. Would you please explain why you rated the care fair/poor?

Not thorough	Quality varies
Inattentive	Unprofessiona

8. How many minutes did you/your family member have to wait before seeing the doctor or APN from the appointment time to when the provider actually met you?

Less than 5 minutes	21–30 minutes
5–10 minutes	Over 30 minutes
11–20 minutes	Don't know

9. How would you rate this APN/doctor on his/her courtesy and friendliness?

Excellent	Fair
Very good	Poor
Good	

10. How would you rate the overall quality of the staff nursing care provided?

Excellent	Fair
Very good	Poor
Good	

11. Would you please explain why you rated the care fair/poor?

Could be better	Quality varies

12. How would you rate the nurses on their courtesy and friendliness?

Excellent	Fair
Very good	Poor
Good	

13. Did you/your family member have any lab tests done—for
    example, blood drawn?
    Yes   No

14. How would you rate that experience?
    Excellent   Fair
    Very good   Poor
    Good

15. Did you/your family member have any radiology tests done, such
    as x rays?
    Yes   No

16. How would you rate that experience?
    Excellent   Fair
    Very good   Poor
    Good

17. Were your/your family member's medication instructions clearly
    written and explained to you/your family member?
    Yes   No

18. Were you/your family member given clear discharge and follow-
    up instructions in writing?
    Yes   No

19. Was your/your family member's bill clear and understandable?
    Yes   No

20. Upon arrival to this clinic, were you/your family member sent to
    New Accounts?
    Yes   No

21. How would you rate the clerks in New Accounts?
    Excellent   Fair
    Very good   Poor
    Good

22. How would you rate the convenience of the location of this clinic?

    Excellent   Fair
    Very good   Poor
    Good

23. How would you rate the overall cleanliness of this clinic?

    Excellent   Fair
    Very good   Poor
    Good

24. What is the likelihood that you would recommend this clinic to your friends or relatives?

    Excellent   Fair
    Very good   Poor
    Good

25. What could this clinic do to improve its services to the community? (Circle all applicable items.)

Nothing	Longer hours
Don't know	Listen to patient/family
Thorough care	Better billing
Prompt provider care	Friendly/caring doctors
More providers	More locations
Better provider availability	Better quality doctors
More staff	Prompt care
Lower costs	Separate waiting area for
Faster test results	children
More convenient location	Prompt ambulance service

North Mississippi Health Services Patient Survey, Family Medical Clinic of Oxford, Oxford, Mississippi, 2002.

Leadership
Self-Assessment

Do you have the qualities to become a valuable leader in your practice?
Review the leadership qualities and ask yourself these questions:

- Attributes
  - ➤ Do I view problems as opportunities?
  - ➤ Do I set priorities?
  - ➤ Do I remain focused?
  - ➤ Am I a creative thinker?
  - ➤ How do I tolerate ambiguity?
  - ➤ Do I portray a positive attitude toward change?
  - ➤ Am I committed to innovations that will improve my practice?

- Skills
  - ➤ Do I clarify my values and beliefs?
  - ➤ Can I inspire and share the vision of my practice?
  - ➤ Can I communicate the strategic business plan for the practice?
  - ➤ Do I recognize realistically the inherent problems in the planning process?
  - ➤ Can I envision the big picture and communicate it to others?
  - ➤ Can I encourage and assist others in the change process?
  - ➤ Do I encourage "reaching the unthinkable" vision?
  - ➤ Can I keep the budget, planning, and policies in line in the practice?
  - ➤ Do I encourage realistic goal setting to reach the vision?
  - ➤ Can I implement realistic plans of action to reach the goals?
  - ➤ Do I communicate the visionary process of planning and change clearly in order to reach attainable practice goals?

- Knowledge
  - ➤ Do I know the responsibilities involved in business planning?
  - ➤ Do I understand the strategic planning process of long- and short-term goals?
  - ➤ Do I understand the practice's vision?
  - ➤ Can I follow the budget aligned for a successful business practice?
  - ➤ Do I understand the factors and barriers that may affect the practice business plan?
  - ➤ Do I know the best methods to achieve the practice's goals?
  - ➤ Do I understand the steps in the process of change and the current paradigm shifts in business and health care systems?
  - ➤ Do I understand the strategies involved in communicating my vision and goals to the community?
  - ➤ Do I involve other members of the practice staff in the decision-making process?
  - ➤ Do I understand what it means to become an advocate for my patients?
  - ➤ Do I understand the best method to resolve conflict with others in the practice and with patients?
  - ➤ Do I understand how to constructively clarify problems and issues and find the appropriate steps of resolution that will build cooperation in promoting joint conflict resolution?

What traits best describe you in the list of questions? Is there any trait that you should consider necessary for your practice that needs attention? If so, where do you go to get the knowledge to improve this trait?

State Positions on Prescriptive Authority for Nurse Practitioners

Independent prescription
(including controlled substances)

Alaska	Maine	New Mexico	Washington
Arizona	Montana	Oregon	Wisconsin
District of Columbia	New Hampshire	Utah*	Wyoming
Iowa			

*Schedule IV and V controlled substances only

Some physician involvement or delegation
(including controlled substances)

Arkansas	Illinois	New York	Maryland
California	Indiana	Ohio	Michigan
Colorado	Kansas	Oklahoma	Minnesota
Connecticut	North Carolina	Pennsylvania	South Dakota
Delaware	North Dakota	Rhode Island	Tennessee
Georgia*	Nebraska	South Carolina*	Virginia
Hawaii	New Jersey	Louisiana	Vermont
Idaho	Nevada	Massachusetts	West Virginia

*Schedule IV and V controlled substances only

Some degree of physician involvement
(excluding controlled substances)

Alabama	Kentucky	Missouri
Florida	Mississippi	Texas

Ethical Decision-Making APN Worksheet

1. Collect facts related to the situation.
   - What are the pertinent facts of the situation—personal, social, interpersonal, psychological, or physical?
   - Is there something wrong in this situation that affects the dignity, rights, and hopes of the patient?
   - Are there health problems, decision needs, or ethical components that go deeper than legal or institutional concerns?

2. Analyze the facts and determine who is involved in making the decision.
   - What individuals are involved in the situation?
   - Who has ownership of the situation?
   - What pertinent relationships are involved in the situation?

3. Clarify issues with the associated ethical principles, theories, laws, and policies.
   - What values are involved in the situation that precipitated the conflict?
   - What is your personal and professional moral position in such a conflict?
   - What are the moral positions of those involved in this conflict?
   - What are the relevant ethical principles, theories, laws, and policies involved in the situation?
   - What interdisciplinary resources can best be utilized in this situation?

4. Interpret the information into a concise statement of the situation.
   - What is the ethical issue pertinent to this situation?

5. Develop a list of actions and their associated projected outcomes.
   - What courses of action can be taken to resolve this situation?
   - What are the probable outcomes of each action?
   - What are the pertinent moral principles involved with each action?
   - What are the projected outcomes when promoting positive moral principles—for example, the most good and the least harm, respect for the rights and dignity of those involved, and fairness for all?

6. Analyze the advantages and disadvantages of the actions.
   - What are the advantages and disadvantages of each action?
   - What guidelines support or invalidate the courses of action?
   - What are the results of similar ethical issues in the applied resources?

7. Identify a plan of action.
   - What is the best plan of action based on your analysis of the situation?

8. Implement the plan.
   - Are you actively participating in the implementation process to ensure conflict resolution?
   - Have the pertinent legal issues governing your scope of practice been applied ?

9. Evaluate the outcome of the plan.
   - Did the implementation of your action result in the outcome projected?
   - If not, what is the best next step to take to resolve the issues?

Quality Health Unlimited: A Sample Strategic Plan

Quality Health Unlimited, PC
Northbrook, IL

Strategic Plan for Operations

Submitted by
Elizabeth Bodie Gross
Elder Link
Barrington, IL

I. Introduction

During the second quarter of 2002, Elder Link consulted with a group of Advanced Practice Nurses (APNs) to determine the viability of developing an APN company that would provide primary care services to residents in skilled nursing facilities (SNFs), assisted living facilities (ALFs), and continuing care retirement communities (CCRCs).

Since this APN company is not seeking outside capitalization, the principals decided that they needed a strategic plan that would outline what activities should be taken during the first fiscal (FY1) four quarters. The following strategic plan has been developed to meet the overall goals and objectives agreed to by the company's principals. They include the following:

- Goals
  - ➤ The company will be positioned as a leader in developing new APN business models.

➢ At the end of the first fiscal year, the company will support two full-time employees (FTEs) and one part-time employee (PTE).
- Objectives
  ➢ Secure five contracts with SNFs, ALFs, and/or CCRCs. (Note: Each contract will ensure 20 hours per week for each APN.)
  ➢ Be pursued by outside interests (e.g., insurance or pharmaceutical companies) to begin marketing and/or presenting the new model to new health care providers.

II. First Quarter FY1

A. *Adopt Business Model*

During the July 2002 meeting, the APN principals voted to adopt the subcontractor model because it is more feasible at this time to establish. This model requires that the company and its clients have a specific set of responsibilities for meeting the objectives outlined previously.

The APN responsibilities include the following:

- Provide monthly invoicing of clients (CCRC/SNF/ALF).
- Provide professional liability for each APN.
- Cover all marketing expenses (e.g., collateral material).
- Pay all of the company's legal and accounting expenses.

Clients are responsible for the following:

- Bill all third-party payers (e.g., Medicare, Medicaid, HMOs, etc.).
- Handle administrative expenses (e.g., office space, equipment, office personnel, supplies, etc.).
- Pay for external marketing expenses/exposure.
- Maintain all client records so that they meet the Health Insurance Portability and Accountability Act (HIPAA) requirements.

B. Company Name

The APN principals voted to adopt one of the following three names:

- Health Perspectives Unlimited, PC
- Quality Health Unlimited, PC
- Experience Health Unlimited, PC

Elder Link has recommended that the name Quality Health Unlimited, PC (hereinafter COMPANY) be chosen since it clearly describes the type of services the company is providing their clients.

Based on the previous recommendation, the following Web site names are available at this time for purchase:

- www.qualityhealthunlimited.com
- www.qualityhealthunlimited.org
- www.qualityhealthunlimited.net
- www.qualityhealthunlimited.us
- www.qualityhealthunlimited.biz

C. Accounting

The COMPANY will secure a contract with an accountant or accounting firm to develop their budgets, ledgers, and accounting systems. If the COMPANY does not subcontract this administrative duty, the accountant/accounting firm will need to train principals on how to maintain appropriate accounting procedures, budgets, ledgers, and so on.

The accountant/accounting firm will also assist the COMPANY in developing pricing strategies so that they meet their first-year goals (Attachment A). The first fiscal year budget has been revised to meet the stated goals and objectives.

D. Administrative

In order for the COMPANY to become operational, several major administrative issues need to be addressed and organized. They include the following:

1. Information Technology

First, the COMPANY needs to acquire appropriate computer systems. This includes, but is not limited to, a desktop computer, laser printer, fax machine, and software that supports operations (e.g., company e-mail, word processing, database, and financial spreadsheets).

Second, the COMPANY needs to secure and develop the specifications for their Web site.

2. Office

First, the COMPANY needs to acquire a centralized post office box. This post office box must be accessible to all APN principals.

Second, the COMPANY needs to set up a central telephone line. The voice mail must be accessible to all APN principals. In addition to setting up the telephone line, it is necessary to develop a schedule for returning and retaining all calls at minimum. Within the development, an APN must check the voice mail at least two times per day (morning and night). Elder Link recommends the voice mail be checked three times per day (morning, noon, and night).

Third, the COMPANY needs to acquire all office equipment (see the previous section "Information Technology"). This includes all furniture and other necessities within the central office.

3. Insurance (Attachments)

- General
- Professional
- Worker's compensation (regulations)

E. Legal

The COMPANY needs to contract a lawyer or law firm to assist them in developing and implementing the following legal instruments:

- Practice agreements
- Investor agreements
- Subcontractor agreements
- Collaborative practice agreements (with physicians)

In addition to the previous elements, legal counsel will review and file all appropriate corporate documentation/forms that are required by the State of Illinois.

Lastly, the COMPANY will consult with either a legal and/or HIPAA consultant on how to comply with the HIPAA regulations. The COMPANY needs to be in compliance by 2003.

F. Marketing and Sales

1. Marketing

First, the COMPANY must secure a contract with a graphic artist to assist the COMPANY in designing their marketing materials.

The contracted graphic artist will develop a logo for the COMPANY that will be printed on all business material (e.g., stationary, business cards, brochures, etc.). Once the logo is developed, the COMPANY will purchase business stationary. This includes, but is not limited, to the following:

- Letterhead
- Envelops
- Business cards

2. Sales

The COMPANY will collaborate with the contracted graphic artist to develop marketing brochures (service offerings) and company folders.

III. Second Quarter FY1

A. Accounting

The office manager/principals will be trained on the accounting systems that have been developed and installed for the COMPANY.

In collaboration with the principals, the contracted accountant/accounting firm will develop accounting policies and procedures for the COMPANY.

B. Administrative

1. Information Technology

In order to develop a Web site, the COMPANY will develop a template that will be used in a Request for Proposal (RFP) for outside vendors. This RFP will outline those activities (and costs) that an outside vendor will perform on the COMPANY's behalf.

Secondly, the COMPANY will continue to develop a policy and procedure manual for the accounting department.

2. Insurance

The COMPANY will continue to review their insurance needs as it expands. This includes, but is not limited to, professional liability, general, and worker's compensation.

C. Legal

As the COMPANY develops their policies and procedures, the legal counsel will also review them to ensure compliance with state regulations. Additionally, the COMPANY needs to develop specific policies and procedures that meet the HIPAA regulations.

D. Marketing and Sales

1. Marketing

The COMPANY will develop marketing templates that specifically target SNFs, ALFs, and CCRCs.

2. Sales

The COMPANY will finalize all marketing materials (e.g., brochures).

IV. Third Quarter FY1

A. Accounting

The COMPANY will finalize all accounting policies and procedures. Also, the COMPANY should begin preparations for their first annual audit.

B. Administration

1. Information Technology

The COMPANY needs to develop an RFP that can be mailed to potential Web site development vendors.

2. Insurance

The COMPANY will continue monitoring all insurance plans to ensure proper coverage for the COMPANY and its employees.

C. Legal

Legal counsel/firm will continue to review all COMPANY policies and procedures, and those specifically designed to meet the HIPAA regulations.

D. Marketing and Sales

1. Marketing

The COMPANY will continue the development of the marketing templates for SNF/ALF/CCRC.

2. Sales

Begin marketing services using new sales templates that respond to RFPs.

V. Fourth Quarter FY1

A. Accounting

The COMPANY prepares and conducts the first-year audit.

B. Administration

1. Information Technology

The COMPANY will review all responses to their RFP and select a vendor. With the vendor's assistance, the Web site development will begin the second fiscal year.

2. Insurance

The COMPANY will continue monitoring all insurance plans to ensure proper coverage for the COMPANY and its employees.

C. Legal

The legal counsel/firm will continue to review all COMPANY policies and procedures, and those specifically designed to meet the HIPAA regulations.

D. Marketing and Sales

1. Marketing

The COMPANY will review marketing materials to determine their effectiveness by developing outcome indicators/measurements.

2. Sales

The COMPANY will review RFP templates and outcome measures (goals) to determine their effectiveness.

Operating Expenses

General and Administrative Expenses	FY1 Q1	FY1 Q2	FY1 Q3	FY1 Q4	YTD FY1
Personnel Expenses					
Salaries*	$40,625	$40,625	$40,625	$40,625	$162,500
Taxes—payroll	$4,672	$4,672	$4,672	$4,672	$18,688
Group insurance benefits					
Consultant expenses					
Total Personnel Expenses	$45,297	$45,297	$45,297	$45,297	$181,188
Office Operations Expenses					
Rent	$0	$0	$0	$0	$0
Taxes—real estate	$0	$0	$0	$0	$0
Commercial insurance	$1,250	$1,250	$1,250	$1,250	$5,000
Utilities	$125	$125	$125	$125	$500
Facility repair and maintenance	$0	$0	$0	$0	$0
Security/fire/alarm	$0	$0	$0	$0	$0
Office equipment—purchase	$250	$250	$250	$250	$1,000
Office equipment—leasing	$250	$250	$250	$250	$1,000
Communications equipment	$250	$250	$250	$250	$1,000
Communications services	$250	$250	$250	$250	$1,000
Information technology equipment	$1,250	$1,250	$1,250	$1,250	$5,000
Information technology software	$250	$250	$250	$250	$1,000
Office furniture	$250	$250	$250	$250	$1,000
Reproduction/printing	$250	$250	$250	$250	$1,000
Postage/package/delivery	$250	$250	$250	$250	$1,000
Licenses/permits	$0	$0	$0	$0	$0
Miscellaneous office expenses	$250	$250	$250	$250	$1,000
Petty cash	$125	$125	$125	$125	$500
Total Office Operations Expenses	$4,750	$4,750	$4,750	$4,750	$19,000

General and Administrative Expenses	FY1 Q1	FY1 Q2	FY1 Q3	FY1 Q4	YTD FY1
Fiscal/Legal Expenses					
Legal expenses	$1,250	$1,250	$1,250	$1,250	$5,000
Accounting services	$1,250	$1,250	$1,250	$1,250	$5,000
Insurance—worker's compensation	$1,250	$1,250	$1,250	$1,250	$5,000
General and professional liability insurance	$625	$625	$625	$625	$2,500
Total Fiscal/Legal Expenses	$4,375	$4,375	$4,375	$4,375	$17,500
Total General and Administrative	$54,422	$54,422	$54,422	$54,422	$217,688
Marketing Expenses					
Conference exhibitions	$125	$125	$125	$125	$500
Graphic artist	$625	$625	$625	$625	$2,500
Marketing materials/collateral	$625	$625	$625	$625	$2,500
Total Marketing Expenses	$1,375	$1,375	$1,375	$1,375	$5,500
Total Operations Expenses	$55,797	$55,797	$55,797	$55,797	$223,188

* The average APN's salary is $65,000.

Time Out for Wellness: A Sample Business Plan

Joni Thanavaro

Executive Summary

Time Out for Wellness, Inc. is an S corporation established in 2002 by Joni Thanavaro, the sole proprietor and owner. The focus of the center is to provide education for health promotion and the prevention of coronary artery disease. Coronary artery disease is the number-one killer of both men and women in the United States. It is estimated that 85% of all cases of coronary artery disease are preventable by using appropriate lifestyle strategies. A recent American Heart Association survey (2000) highlights how more and more Americans are concerned about coronary artery disease risk factors and are seeking assistance with developing strategies to help reduce their risks.

The center will be located in Town and Country, Missouri, in an office-building suite in an area zoned for medical care. The center is located within 1 mile of two level-I hospitals. The office suite is newly remodeled and is available for immediate occupancy. Currently, there is a lack of high-quality specialized services directed toward the health care promotion needs of middle-aged and older adults in this geographic area.

The target population for the center is men and women between the ages of 45 and 60 since they are at the highest risk for coronary artery disease. The median age of the population of Town and Country and the surrounding suburbs fits this demographic. Research-supported strategies, known to reduce coronary artery risk, including smoking cessation, exercise, diet and weight management, and stress reduction programs will be the cornerstones of the services provided at the center. Product lines and additional services including blood and exercise testing will be added on once the center is established.

The popular culture of the Town and Country area has demonstrated a consistent willingness to seek out and embrace services when they perceive these services will enhance their well being. The number of dollars spent annually for such out-of-pocket health care and promotion services is evidence of this.

Time Out for Wellness, Inc. will offer products and services that do not exist in any one location anywhere in the greater St. Louis area. All services provided will be directed and taught by Advanced Practice Nurses (APNs) who are board certified and who have experience in working with and meeting the needs of customers seeking risk factor modification strategies. All services will be paid directly by the consumer.

Vision Statement

Time Out for Wellness, Inc. promotes comprehensive lifestyle strategies for optimum health.

Values

At Time Out for Wellness, Inc., we believe that our business should be based on a high quality of care that is

- Customer satisfaction driven
- Community oriented
- Holistic

Mission Statement

Time Out for Wellness, Inc. provides individualized education to influence positive heart-healthy choices.

Mission Goals

- To provide a wide range of risk factor modification programs for the targeted population

- To be proactive in promoting healthy lifestyle practices in the community

Operational Goals

First Year

- To establish a successful business that will be profitable by the end of the first year of operation
- To provide a minimum of 36 visits a week by the end of 3 months of operation
- To have a minimum of 72 visits a week by the end of 6 months of operation
- To reach full capacity with 140 visits a week by the end of the first year of operation
- To provide a select line of vitamins, books, and exercise monitors
- To establish a Web site and on-site library for customers by the end of 6 months of operation
- To establish a cooperative relationship with insurance companies, major local corporations, and fitness programs for referrals, and area businesses for advertising and marketing

Second Year

- To remain profitable with a 20% increase in profit margin
- To increase sales of product lines by 5%

Third Year

- To establish additional diagnostic screening including lipid profiles, blood sugars, EKGs, and stress testing
- To add additional staff and increase customer visits

Organizational Plan

Description of the Business

Time Out for Wellness, Inc. is a unique company that will provide services to men and women over the age of 18 who are interested in reducing their risks of cardiovascular disease by lifestyle modification. Currently, there is no such business in the area providing these services in a comprehensive manner. Numerous health care and freestanding companies in the area provide portions of the services proposed. However, Time Out for Wellness, Inc. will provide high-quality and comprehensive services that are currently unavailable. The company will be housed in a 2,000-square-foot office building suite at the corner of Ballas and Clayton Roads in Town and Country.

Products and Services

Time Out for Wellness, Inc. will provide a comprehensive range of risk factor modification programs that are directed toward primary health promotion. Individual counseling will be offered in 1-hour time periods and will be given by APNs who are board certified.

The Wellness Center's environment is designed to create a space that is comfortable and welcoming. All customers will have their blood pressures and weight taken and tracked at each visit.

A continuous quality improvement (CQI) process will be utilized to evaluate and maintain the highest quality for all services provided. New programs will be added as the needs are identified.

The list of programs being offered include the following:

- **Smoking cessation**   A 7- to 12-week program based on the individual needs of the customer
- **Stress management**   A 12-week initial program with provisions to extend the duration of sessions based on the needs of the customer
- **Diet and weight management**   A 12-week initial program that can also be extended as needed
- **Exercise management**   A 4-week initial program to prepare the customer for safe and effective exercise
- **Support groups**   Offered for all programs

Product Lines

- **Vitamins**   A wide variety of which research has shown to decrease the risk of coronary artery disease including Vitamin B and C complex, Vitamin E, folic acid, and Omega-3 fatty acids

- **Exercise monitors**   A variety of high-quality monitors to provide heart rates and distance guides while exercising

Library

- Books for further learning for all program content
- Audio books
- Videos

Time Out for Wellness Web Site

- An ask-the-nurse site for questions and answers
- Monthly tips on strategies to promote healthy lifestyles
- Recipe of the month

Management and Personnel

Time Out for Wellness, Inc. will be managed by Joni Thanavaro, a board-certified nurse practitioner with a master's degree in cardiovascular nursing. Thanavaro has extensive nursing experience caring for healthy adults as well as those with heart disease. Since she has worked in the Town and Country area for 15 years, she has established numerous contacts and relationships within the community. She is deeply committed to teaching customers how to modify their risks for developing heart disease. Additional full-time personnel will include three APNs and an administrative assistant.

Organizational Structure

Time Out for Wellness, Inc. is a corporation that operates using a matrix structure. The APNs and the administrative assistant report directly to the director. The health advisory board reviews standards of care and best practice strategies with the adult nurse practitioners. The health advisory board is made up of the following:

- Two adult nurse practitioners from St. Louis University
- One primary care physician
- One cardiologist
- One consumer

A collaborating physician serves in a consulting role. The organizational chart is as follows.

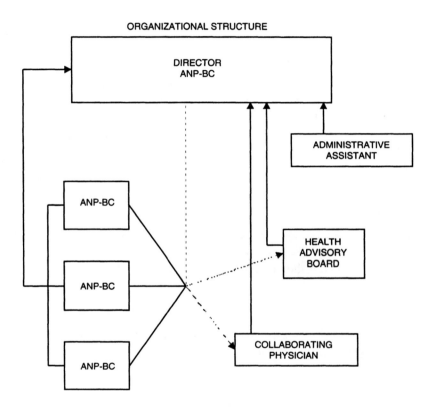

ORGANIZATIONAL STRUCTURE

DIRECTOR
ANP-BC

ADMINISTRATIVE
ASSISTANT

ANP-BC

HEALTH
ADVISORY
BOARD

ANP-BC

ANP-BC

COLLABORATING
PHYSICIAN

Legal Structure

Based on recommendations of Phillip Kaplan, Attorney at Law, Time Out for Wellness, Inc. will be established as a subchapter S corporation. The corporation establishment process has begun and corporation status by the State of Missouri is pending. The name and logo of Time Out for Wellness, Inc. will be registered and trademarked according to the law of the State of Missouri. The Web site address of Time Out for Wellness, Inc. will be registered as www.timeoutforwellness.com.

Location

Time Out for Wellness, Inc. is located in one of the most affluent areas in the United States. The long-standing cultural normal will be an active consumer of luxury indulgences.

Accounting and Record Keeping

Time Out for Wellness, Inc. has contracted Sexton and Associates for the corporation's accounting needs. The administrative assistant will maintain records of all receipts and will prepare reports as mandated by the accountant. The administrative assistant is responsible for inputting all client data and maintaining current records. Financial auditing will be done monthly by the contracted accountant.

Insurance

All professional staff will be responsible for holding professional liability insurance as well as maintaining the current certification and licensure. Copies of the current policies will be kept on file.

Summary

Time Out for Wellness, Inc. will offer services that currently do not exist in this area for health promotion.

Marketing Plan

Target Market

The following demographic information has been obtained through a comprehensive market analysis performed by Demographics (2000 MSA Demographic Information).

- County of Town and Country
  - ➤ Economic level: middle to upper class
  - ➤ Income level: $140,000+ annual income
  - ➤ Median age: 45 to 60

➢ Educational level: 22% graduate or professional degree
39% associate/bachelor's degree
20% some college
➢ Employment rate: 2.2% unemployed
➢ Race: 93.4% White
2.2% Black
4.0% Asian
1.4% Hispanic
➢ Psychological makeup: concerned with health and well being
➢ Habits: consumers of high-quality specialized services who enjoy engaging in leisure-time activities
➢ Shop: specialty boutiques offering unique, high-quality, and high-priced products, and a high usage of vitamins and supplements (65% of all consumers surveyed)
➢ Market size: population 20,053

Competition

The main competitors for this business are as follows:

- One fitness center, 10 miles from Time Out for Wellness, Inc., that offers nonindividualized group exercise programs
- One hospital, 1 mile from Time Out for Wellness, Inc., that has dieticians on staff for diet and weight management counseling

Both competitors offer only one of the services provided at Time Out for Wellness, Inc. The fitness center has no provision for one-on-one instruction for an exercise program. The hospital provides diet instruction in an impersonal hospital environment versus the comfortable and friendly environment of Time Out for Wellness, Inc.

Methods of Distribution

All services and products will be offered on site.

Promotion

The marketing objectives are to initiate a heavy campaign primarily to position Time Out for Wellness, Inc. as a community social center as well as the premiere location for personalized assistance with healthy lifestyle practices. Strategies will include the following.

Publicity

- Feature articles in the *Ladue News*
- Feature articles in the *St. Louis Post-Dispatch*
- Ten-minute TV time slot on *Show Me St. Louis*

Paid Advertising

- Six-month advertisement in *St. Louis Business Magazine*

Directory Listings

- St. Louis County area White Pages (one line)
- St. Louis County area Yellow Pages (two lines)
- Local Yellow Pages (one-fourth page)

Distribution of Printed Material

Promotional fliers are mailed to the following:

- Local grocery, drug, and exercise stores
- Every household in Town and Country and the surrounding suburbs

Open House

- On-premises open house (potential customers will be able to tour the center)
- Local celebrities to promote healthy lifestyle choices
- Wine and cheese as refreshments

Pricing

All customers receive free blood pressure and weight monitoring for each visit:

- **Smoking cessation.** $75 a visit. A 7- to 12-week program that can extended if needed.

- **Stress management.** $150 a visit. A 12-week program that can be extended if needed. Reenrollment of some customers is anticipated.
- **Diet and weight management.** $150 a visit. A 12-week program that can be extended, if needed. Reenrollment of some customers is anticipated.
- **Exercise management.** $75 a visit. A 4-week program that can be extended if needed.
- **Support groups.**   Offered on a weekly basis free of charge for each of the previous programs.
- **Vitamins.**   Sold at 20% above the market price.
  - ➤ Folic acid
  - ➤ Vitamin E
  - ➤ Omega-3 fatty acids
  - ➤ B complex
  - ➤ C complex
- **Books and exercise monitors.**   Sold at 20% above the market price.

Environmental Design

Time Out for Wellness, Inc. resides in a 2,000-square-foot office suite at Ballas and Clayton Roads. It consists of four counseling rooms, a reception area, and a waiting room. There are two restroom facilities. The interior of all rooms will be furnished with high-quality furniture. The reception area and waiting room will be designed with attention to elegance and comfort. Products for sale will be displayed in one corner of the reception area. The exterior is beautifully landscaped and has ample parking space.

Hours of Operation

The hours of operation for Time Out for Wellness, Inc. will be Monday through Friday from 9 a.m. to 5 p.m.

Support classes will be held one evening a week as follows:

- Smoking cessation support group: Monday, 7:00 to 8:30 p.m.
- Stress reduction support group: Tuesday, 7:00 to 8:30 p.m.

- Diet and weight management support group: Wednesday, 7:00 to 8:30 p.m.
- Exercise support group: Thursday, 7:00 to 8:30 p.m.

After 1 year, it is anticipated that weekend hours will be offered. The director will be available by beeper every evening until 10 p.m.

Timing of Market Entry

The clinical, organizational, and operational timelines for the center can be found in the "Support Documents" section of this business plan. The recent untimely death of St. Louis Cardinal baseball star Daryl Kile, at the age of 33, to coronary artery disease is likely to have a critical impact on the perceived magnitude of this illness in the community. Invitations for the grand opening, scheduled for Saturday, December 7, will be mailed out in early November. St. Louis Cardinal baseball players will be recruited to be present for the opening in honor of Daryl Kile.

Financial Documents

Summary of Financial Needs

Time Out for Wellness, Inc. is seeking a $100,000 loan to cover the following:

- The purchase of equipment and supplies
- The purchase of furniture
- Offset projected losses in the first 6 months

Loan Fund Dispersal Statement

A portion of the loan amount will be used to purchase equipment and supplies, and the remainder of the loan will be used to cover expenses and meet payroll during the first 6 months of operation. A detailed summary of the total start-up fees can be found in the "Supporting Documents" section of this business plan.

Job Descriptions

Job Description for the Director

Duties include, but are not limited to, the following:

- Oversee the general day-to-day activities of the center.
- Troubleshoot customer complaints or concerns.
- Maintain financial reports.
- Perform employee evaluations.
- Schedule and conduct monthly staff meetings with staff.
- Schedule and conduct quarterly meetings with the health advisory board.
- Provide counseling to consumers.
- Document the progress of each visit.

Job Description for the APNs

Duties include, but are not limited to, the following:

- Develop and update patient education materials.
- Develop and maintain the Web site.
- Provide counseling to consumers.
- Document the progress of consumers at each visit.
- Make referrals, as needed, to health care providers.

Job Description for the Administrative Assistant

Duties include, but are not limited to, the following:

- Schedule visits.
- Receive and document payment for visits.
- Accompany customers to counseling rooms.
- Order supplies and product lines.
- Sell products to consumers.

Supporting Documents

Timelines

Clinical Timeline

Task	Target Date	Completed
Write standards of care.	July 1, 2002	
Begin interviewing for staff.	August 1, 2002	
Hire three APNs and an administrative assistant.	November 1, 2002	
Start training on the computer.	December 1, 2002	
First date to see customers.	January 2, 2003	
Nine customers seen weekly.	January–March 2003	
Eighteen customers seen weekly.	April–June 2003	
Twenty-seven customers seen weekly.	July–September 2003	
Thirty-five customers seen weekly.	October–December 2003	
Conduct performance evaluations.	June 2003	
Conduct quality standards evaluations.	June 2003	

Operational Timeline

Task	Target Date	Completed
Order supplies.	October 1, 2002	
Buy furniture.	October 30, 2002	
Buy computers.	November 10, 2002	
Arrange for utilities, cable, and phone lines.	November 20, 2002	
Prepare treatment rooms.	December 1, 2002	

Organizational Timeline

Task	Target Date	Completed
Develop organizational chart.	July 1, 2002	
Develop policies and procedures.	August 1, 2002	
Place ads.	September 1, 2002	
Develop marketing materials.	September 15, 2002	
Seek out potential shareholders.	September 30, 2002	
Apply for loan.	October 15, 2002	
Plan open house.	October 30, 2002	

Start-up Fees

Start-up Fees	Amount
Attorney—incorporation fee	$1,700
Furniture—treatment rooms	$10,000
Furniture—reception and waiting area	$10,000
Six phones	$500
Installation costs	$500
Five computers	$7,500
Two laser printers	$1,600
Copier/fax	$400
Blood pressure cuffs and scale	$1,000
Cell phones, beepers, and palm pilots	$3,000
Stereo system	$1,400
VCR, TV, and cart	$600
Marketing fees	$10,000
Total Start-up Costs	**$48,200**

Total Yearly Expenses

Expenses	Amount
Direct Expenses	
Salaries (four APNs)	$250,000
Administrative assistant	$25,000
Benefits (30%) (includes taxes)	$75,000
Continuing education	$10,000
Total Direct Expenses	**$310,000**
Indirect Expenses	
Loan repayment (5 years at 8%)	$24,800
Phone ($400 a month)	$4,800
Electric ($500 a month)	$6,000
Internet ($40 a month)	$480
Accountant (payroll—$200 a month)	$2,400
Housekeeping ($400 a month)	$4,800
Rent ($20 a square foot for 2,000 square feet)	$40,000
Paper	$2,500
Mailing	$3,000
Business cards	$300
Total Indirect Expenses	**$89,080**
Total Yearly Expenses	**$399,080**

Summary for Expenses and Revenues

	2003 Jan.–Mar.	2003 Apr.–June	2003 July–Sept.	2003 Oct.–Dec.	2004 Annual	2005 Annual
Expenses	$99,770	$99,770	$99,770	$99,770	419,000	439,984
Revenues						
Customer visits	$47,000	$95,000	$142,000	$189,000	$756,000	$756,000
Product sales	$960	$1,320	$2,880	$3,840	$16,128	$16,932
Total revenue	$47,960	$96,320	$144,880	$192,640	$772,126	$772,932
Cumulative revenues	$51,810	$55,260	$10,150	$82,920	$353,128	$332,946

Greenup Well Family Care Center: A Business Plan

Anita England
Nancy Fagan
Barbara Henrichon
Barbra Keller
Jeani Thomas

Executive Summary

Greenup Well Family Care Center is an S corporation established in 2001 to provide health care services to all ages. Although the focus of the center is to provide primary care, services will be available to care for individuals with minor acute problems. The clinic is located on Route 23 in the city of Greenup, Kentucky. The center is newly remodeled, handicapped accessible, equipped for a medical practice, and available for immediate occupancy. This site was chosen based on a needs assessment completed by the Greenup Chamber of Commerce. Currently, there is only one physician within a 10-mile radius; he is scheduled to retire in 5 years and is no longer accepting new patients. The nearest hospital is located 16 miles away.

The clinic is committed to providing high-quality, cost-effective health care in a warm and inviting atmosphere. The focus of the practice is on prevention and wellness, while providing the evaluation and treatment of acute and chronic diseases.

The corporation consists of five Advanced Practice Nurses (APNs), who in addition to caring for patients, will oversee the day-to-day operation of the clinic. Résumés of the APN stockholders can be found in

Appendix A. APNs perform physical examinations; record medical, family, and psychosocial histories; direct and implement health promotion and therapeutic regimens; and prescribe medications. The APNs will donate their time for the first year to facilitate growth in the corporation. The clinic will have three paid employees. The receptionist, a full-time employee, will be recruited from the community. This position will require someone with experience in a health care facility. The receptionist will provide a valuable link to the community. A full-time LPN will function as office manager with responsibilities for scheduling and overseeing the patient flow. A collaborating physician will be retained as a resource person and assume the care of patients who are in need of hospitalization or procedures not in the APNs' scope of practice.

The clinic's target population will include clients of all ages, families, local business workers, and health insurers. Aggressive marketing will include local advertising through TV, radio, and newspaper ads, direct mailings, participation in community events, and health fairs. An open house offering free blood pressure screenings will start the campaign. This gives community members the opportunity to visit the clinic as well as meet the health care providers. The open house is scheduled for January 2, 2002. Patients will be scheduled as of January 5, 2002.

The clinic has four exam rooms that will accommodate two practitioners as business increases. Patient volume is estimated to be 20 patients per day for the first year with an expected growth of 10% each year following.

A line of credit of $100,000 will be needed for start-up costs and operating expenses for the first year until incoming revenues meet the needs of the clinic. Fifty percent of the loan will be needed to open the business, with 25% at the end of the first month and 25% percent at the end of the second month. The break-even point is projected at the end of the third month. The repayment of the loan and interest can begin promptly within 30 days of receiving funds. The projected income for the first year is $201,000. The total operating expenses are projected at $108,000 for the first year. This will leave an operating income of $93,000. These funds will be used toward paying outstanding loans and reinvesting in the business. Each of the five stockholders will place a $20,000 certificate of deposit in escrow as collateral for this loan.

Company Overview and Description

Mission Statement

Greenup Well Family Care Center is committed to excellence, providing high-quality, cost-effective health care to persons of all ages. Although our goal is to serve as primary care providers, we also care for minor problems.

Values

At Greenup Well Family Care Center, we believe that above all else our business should be based on high-quality care that is

- Community oriented
- Customer satisfaction driven
- Holistic
- Cost effective
- Accessible
- Nondiscriminatory

Corporate Vision Statement

Greenup Well Family Care Center aspires to gain a local reputation as being one of the best health care providers in the city.

Corporation

Greenup Well Family Care Center is organized as a corporation. The organization is created by a government charter, which enables the health care providers to associate together for a common purpose under a common name. The charter gives the corporation certain privileges, including the right to buy and sell property, enter into contracts, sue and be sued, and borrow and lend money. The care center is a private corporation, which means that it is founded and owned by a small group of individuals—the health care providers.

Organizing as a corporation offers the Greenup Well Family Care Center certain advantages. The owners of the corporation enjoy limited liability—that is, they are not liable for the corporation's debts. If the corporation discontinues business, its creditors have a claim only on the assets of the corporation, not on the personal assets of its owners. Another advantage of a corporation is its ability to raise vast amounts of capital. By issuing stock, a corporation can enable thousands of individuals to pool financial resources and invest in a new venture. This also spreads the risk of financial loss among many people. In the beginning phases of the corporation, stock will not be for sale to the general public. However, as the business grows, offering stock may become a reality.

Organizational Structure

Greenup Well Family Care Center is a corporation that operates using a matrix structure. The corporation is ready for change, competitive, and diverse, and maintains high standards and social responsibility. The care center is organic in nature and provides an informal, decentralized environment. A few departments offer large amounts of rich information, experience, and technical knowledge through boundary spanning. The flexible sharing of human resources across products and services provides the motivation, commitment, and opportunity for development.

The organizational chart is as follows.

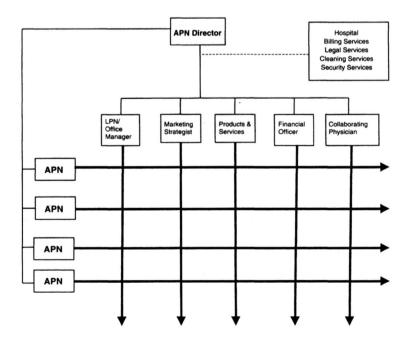

Marketing Strategy

Objective

The initial objective is to promote and support services provided by the Greenup Well Family Care Center as convenient and superior to those currently available while treating each client as a long-term customer. In order to achieve this goal, the overall marketing plan will be based on three fundamentals:

1. Targeting a segment of the population
2. Selecting distribution channels to reach the target market
3. Capturing a share of the market

Ads and Promotion

The marketing objective is to initiate a heavy campaign primarily to position the corporation as the health care provider of choice in the Greenup community. The ads and promotion campaign will require extensive, wide-based promotion to ensure service recognition. Strategies include the following:

- Yellow Page ads.
- Press releases.
- News articles.
- Business cards and flyers.
- Letterhead stationary.
- Local cable television ads.
- Promotional fact sheets suitable for distribution.
- Flyers/brochures and posters for distribution at local senior centers, libraries, rest stops on major highways, local major attractions, and campgrounds.
- Ads and repetitive appearances on local radio broadcasts.
- Lunch meetings with prominent local leaders for one-on-one promotion.
- Formal presentations to local civic groups, athletic clubs, chambers of commerce, and senior centers.
- Future promotions will include community education workshops, an ongoing health-related newspaper column, and Web site.

- Public relations will continue with appearances at civic meetings, television and radio programs, and community events, and membership in local organizations to establish and maintain a presence in the community.

Media Campaign

The Greenup Well Family Care Center will gain public awareness of the services provided. Media promotion will establish an image of caring, reliable, and easily accessible professionals. It will be important to schedule a media campaign with adequate frequency to impact the local market with a positive corporate image and superior services. This campaign will focus on a targeted audience consisting of families and tourists while getting the most out of our promotional budget.

Ad Campaign

The delivery and tone of the advertising will convey the look and feel of professional efficiency, be attractive, and feel comfortable. Advertising must address any known or anticipated corporate objectives, and be consistent and easy to understand based on the reading level of the target audience. Ads will convey factual messages promoting a superior product. These messages will be conveyed through endorsements from community leaders, testimonials from customers, and the presentations of facts about the organization and the people behind it.

Incentives

Incentives offered to customers of the care center will include coffee mugs, refrigerator magnets, pens, and t-shirts with the corporation's logo all aimed at name recognition and keeping the corporation's name in front of the customer. Company-sponsored blood pressure and other health screenings will link the corporation's name with health promotion.

Direct Mail

A direct mail campaign to advertise the open house will help to generate customers.

Customer Service

Customer service will address the consumer's concerns with health care accessibility should a medical emergency arise during off-hours. The clinic will promote 24-hour phone accessibility to address health care needs. Other strategies will include the acceptance of all insurances, credit cards, and an available sliding scale payment plan.

Packaging

A strict professional dress code will be incorporated for all employees. The storefront, waiting room, and examination rooms will incorporate furniture and decorations that will continue to convey the corporate image of professionalism along with comfort and care.

Analysis of the Market

We intend to reach prospective customers in the Greenup County area. Currently, one local physician and two hospitals within a 20-mile radius share the market. The stability of the market is expected to change with the retirement of the local physician within the next 2 years.

Strengths

The corporation's most powerful asset will be our prominent presence in the community.

Weaknesses

There are currently no environmental threats of concern.

Location

The proposed location of the Well Family Care Center was chosen for the following reasons:

- Availability
- Central location

- Ease of accessibility via public and private transportation
- Visibility
- Ease and low cost of conversion to a workable space

Greenup is in the eastern coal field region of Kentucky. Country Music Highway U.S. 23 is a scenic drive featuring a heritage of famous eastern Kentucky music stars.

Population Density

The following is information collected from the 1990 census for the city of Greenup:

- Number of families: 505
- 2.02 sq. km
- 118 miles to the state capital

Demographics (1995 MSA Demographic Information)

Greenup County has the following demographics:

- Median household income: $21,296
- Mean household income: $27,912
- Median age: 37.4
- Race: 96% White, 10% Black, and 10% Hispanic
- Education
  - ➤ Completed grade 9 or less: 15%
  - ➤ Completed grades 9–12: 18%
  - ➤ High school graduate: 35%
  - ➤ Some college: 15%
  - ➤ Have an undergraduate degree: less than 5%
  - ➤ Have a graduate degree: less than 5%
- Employment
  - ➤ Unemployment rate: 6.6%
  - ➤ Citizens who fall below the poverty level (1993 demographics): 18.3%

Additional demographics are available in Appendix B.

The following individuals will make up the customer base of the clinic:

- Children/adolescents
- Adults
- Seniors
- Families
- Clients with chronic illnesses (diabetes, hypertension, etc.)
- Clients with acute minor illnesses
- Small business owners
- Farmers
- Migrant workers
- Small industry laborers (local steel mill workers)
- Truckers
- Schools
- Railroad laborers (CSX Railroad)
- Tourists
- Local business workers (firemen, police, coal miners, local unions, ambulance workers, etc.)
- Social Services (HHS office)
- Health insurers

Competition

Competition can be expected from two key areas:

- Within a 10-mile radius, there is one local physician. This physician is scheduled to retire within 5 years and is no longer accepting new clients.
- The nearest hospital/health care centers are located 16 miles east and 20 miles west.

Other Influences

- The hospital satellite clinic in Greenup is scheduled to close within the next 2 years due to nonprofitability. The satellite clinic offered restricted hours and services and was not adequately promoted in the community.

- The satellite center was newly remolded within the last 18 months and is fully equipped for a medical practice.
- The satellite center is located within a strip mall in the center of town.
- The satellite center has ample parking and is handicapped accessible.
- The satellite center is available for lease.
- A pharmacy is located within the strip mall for easy customer access.

Services of the Greenup Well Family Care Center

The Greenup Well Family Care Center offers an alternative choice in premier primary care by nurse practitioners. A nurse practitioner is a master's prepared registered nurse who has received additional education, training, and certification, and is qualified to provide primary patient care. Nurse practitioners collaborate with physicians and other health care personnel. Nurse practitioners specialize in providing health care across the continuum of the life span. The nurse practitioner partners at the center are actively involved in the community through volunteerism and coalition building with other community organizations and community members. Continued support of the nursing profession by the nurse practitioner partners is provided through leadership of professional nursing organizations providing preceptorship to APN students.

Services provided by the nurse practitioner partners are in compliance with the Kentucky Board of Nursing "scope and standards of practice of advanced registered nurse practitioners" 201 KAR 20:057 and is governed by the Advanced Registered Nurse Practice Council. There is a collaborative practice agreement with a physician, which defines the scope of prescriptive authority. It also delineates the areas of practice with an established protocol for seeking consultation or referral in those situations outside the advanced registered nurse practitioner's scope of practice. The nurse practitioner partners jointly approved the agreement along with the collaborative physician in accordance with the statutory authority KRS 314.131(1) of the Kentucky Board of Nursing.

Competitive Advantage

The Greenup Well Family Care Center will provide evening and week-end hours along with a daily appointment schedule. Walk-in appointments will also be available. The Greenup Well Family Care Center will have a nurse practitioner available to the patients of the Greenup Well Family Care Center 24 hours by telephone for their urgent health care needs.

Nurse practitioners at the Greenup Well Family Care Center provide a variety of services, such as the following:

- Obtain medical, family, and psychosocial histories.
- Perform physical exams: annual, sports, DOT, and pelvic exams.
- Order and interpret diagnostic studies.
- Diagnose and treat common health problems and minor injuries.
- Diagnose, treat, and monitor chronic diseases such as arthritis, diabetes, and hypertension.
- Prescribe medications and treatments.
- Provide family planning services.
- Provide well-child checks including immunizations, growth monitoring, immunizations, and provide anticipatory guidance.
- Educate patients and the community concerning positive health behaviors that promote health and wellness.
- Provide education on weight management, nutrition, and smoking cessation.
- Promote health and wellness within the community by participating in screening programs and educational activities.
- Work with physicians and other health care providers to provide multidisciplinary health services.
- Treat minor podiatry procedures such as toenail and corn removal.
- Suture minor lacerations.
- Splint minor fractures.
- Provide birth control methods, screen for and treat sexually transmitted diseases, and perform Pap smears.
- Perform a colposcopy with or without biopsy.

- Provide walk-in care services for anyone needing care for minor injuries or acute illnesses.

The following laboratory tests will be provided:

- Rapid testing for strep infection
- Urine dip stick or tablet analysis of urine
- Fecal occult blood analysis
- Wet mount and KOH examination of fluids from pelvic exams
- Quick flu testing

The 5-Year Projection

The Greenup Well Family Care Center projects that by the end of the fifth operating year, the following goals will be realized:

- Debt free
- Two full-time salaried providers each day
- In-house billing
- Additional services (home visits for homebound and elderly, and occupational health)
- Extended hours
- Benefits/retirement for all employees
- Continued growth (10% a year)

Income Statement—12 Months

Period Starting	Month 1	Month 2	Month 3	Month 4	Month 5	Month 6	Month 7	Month 8	Month 9	Month 10	Month 11	Month 12	Totals
Charges													
Medicare—30%	8,610	7,890	8,250	7,890	8,610	7,890	8,250	8,610	7,530	8,610	7,890	7,530	97,560
Medicaid—50%	14,360	13,110	13,750	13,110	14,360	13,110	13,750	14,360	12,500	14,360	13,110	12,500	162,380
Insurance—10%	2,860	2,640	2,750	2,640	2,860	2,640	2,750	2,860	2,500	2,860	2,640	2,500	32,500
Self-pay—10%	2,860	2,640	2,750	2,640	2,860	2,640	2,750	2,860	2,500	2,860	2,640	2,500	32,500
Total Charges	28,690	26,280	27,500	26,280	28,690	26,280	27,500	28,690	25,030	28,690	26,280	25,030	324,940
Less Contractual Allowances													
Medicare	3,444	3,156	3,300	3,156	3,444	3,156	3,300	3,444	3,012	3,444	3,156	3,012	39,024
Medicaid	5,744	5,244	5,500	5,244	5,744	5,244	5,500	5,744	5,000	5,744	5,244	5,000	64,952
Insurance	286	264	275	264	286	264	275	286	250	286	264	250	3,250
Self-pay	1,430	1,320	1,375	1,320	1,430	1,320	1,375	1,430	1,250	1,430	1,320	1,250	16,250
Total Cost of Goods Sold	10,904	9,984	10,450	9,984	10,904	9,984	10,450	10,904	9,512	10,904	9,984	9,512	123,476
Gross profit	17,786	16,296	17,050	16,296	17,786	16,296	17,050	17,786	15,518	17,786	16,296	15,518	201,464
Operating Expenses													
Salaries and wages	3,000	3,000	3,000	3,000	3,000	3,000	3,000	3,000	3,000	3,000	3,000	3,000	36,000
Employee benefits	400	400	400	400	400	400	400	400	400	400	400	400	4,800
Payroll taxes	250	250	250	250	250	250	250	250	250	250	250	250	3,000
Rent	1,000	1,000	1,000	1,000	1,000	1,000	1,000	1,000	1,000	1,000	1,000	1,000	12,000
Utilities	500	500	500	500	500	500	500	500	500	500	500	500	6,000

	Period Starting	Month 1	Month 2	Month 3	Month 4	Month 5	Month 6	Month 7	Month 8	Month 9	Month 10	Month 11	Month 12	Totals
Malpractice insurance	3,500													3,500
Liability insurance	500													500
Billing	460	420	440	420	460	420	440	460	400	460	420	400		5,200
Telephone	500	500	500	500	500	500	500	500	500	500	500	500		6,000
Postage	30	30	30	30	30	30	30	30	30	30	30	30		360
Office supplies	100	100	100	100	100	100	100	100	100	100	100	100		1,200
Disposable supplies	150	150	150	150	150	150	150	150	150	150	150	150		1,800
Printing	300				50			50				50		450
Advertising	700				100		100			300				1,200

Income Statement—12 Months

	Period Starting	Month 1	Month 2	Month 3	Month 4	Month 5	Month 6	Month 7	Month 8	Month 9	Month 10	Month 11	Month 12	Totals
Answering service	75	75	75	75	75	75	75	75	75	75	75	75		900
Professional fees			750			750			750			750		3,000
Cleaning/snow removal	260	160	160	160	160	160	160	160	160	160	160	260		2,120
Bank charges	50	50	50	50	50	50	50	50	50	50	50	50		600
Loan payment	1,500	1,500	1,500	1,500	1,500	1,500	1,500	1,500	1,500	1,500	1,500	1,500		18,000
Petty cash	50	50	50	50	50	50	50	50	50	50	50	50		600
Accounting				200				100		100				400
Legal fees	600	50	50	50	50	50	50	50	50	50	50	50		1,150
Security service	100	100	100	100	100	100	100	100	100	100	100	100		1,200
Total Operating Expenses	14,025	8,335	9,105	8,535	8,525	9,085	8,455	8,525	9,065	8,775	8,335	9,215		109,980

(continued)

Financial Review/Budget (continued)

Period Starting	Month 1	Month 2	Month 3	Month 4	Month 5	Month 6	Month 7	Month 8	Month 9	Month 10	Month 11	Month 12	Totals
Operating income	3,761	7,961	7,945	7,761	9,261	7,211	8,595	9,261	6,453	9,011	7,961	6,303	91,484
Interest income (expense)	0	0	0	0	0	0	0	0	0	0	0	0	0
Other income (expense)	0	0	0	0	0	0	0	0	0	0	0	0	0
Total nonoperating income (expense)	0	0	0	0	0	0	0	0	0	0	0	0	0
Income (loss) before taxes	3,761	7,961	7,945	7,761	9,261	7,211	8,595	9,261	6,453	9,011	7,961	6,303	91,484
Income taxes													
Net income (loss)	3,761	7,961	7,945	7,761	9,261	7,211	8,595	9,261	6,453	9,011	7,961	6,303	91,484
Cumulative Net Income (Loss)	3,761	11,722	19,667	27,428	36,689	43,900	52,495	61,756	68,209	77,220	85,181	91,484	91,484

Business Environment

Boyd and Greenup Counties—Demographics

Population by Age

	Boyd and Greenup Counties		Labor Market Area	
	Number	Percent	Number	Percent
Under 18	18,972	22.2	99,470	23.6
18–24	6,791	7.9	40,533	9.6
25–34	10,376	12.1	51,303	12.2
35–44	13,962	16.3	63,663	15.1
45–54	13,066	15.3	61,823	14.6
55–64	9,497	11.1	43,710	10.4
65–74	7,346	8.6	32,705	7.7
75 and older	5,565	6.5	28,864	6.8
Median age	**40.0**	**38.3**		

Source: U.S. Department of Commerce, Bureau of the Census (1999).

Population by Race and Origin

	Boyd and Greenup Counties		Labor Market Area	
	Number	Percent	Number	Percent
White	84,666	98.0	411,868	97.3
Black	1,262	1.5	9,332	2.2
Asian, Pacific Islander	360	0.4	1,422	0.3
American Indian	129	0.1	886	0.2
Hispanic	696	0.8	2,011	0.5

Source: U.S. Department of Commerce, Bureau of the Census (1999).

Personal Income

	1993	1998	Percent Change
Boyd and Greenup Counties	$18,176	$21,687	19.3
Kentucky	$17,815	$22,183	24.5
United States	$21,718	$27,203	25.3
Labor market area	$11,262–$19,942	$13,495–$23,571	

Source: U.S. Department of Commerce, Bureau Economic Analysis.

Number of Households

	Persons per Household	Median Household Income
19,876	2.5	$32,239

Source: U.S. Department of Commerce, Bureau of the Census.

Boyd and Greenup Counties—Quality of Life

In 1999, the median home price in Boyd County was $60,000.

Climate

Temperature
    Normal (59-year record)   55.7 degrees
    Average annual, 1999   56.6 degrees
    Record highest, July 1988 (39-year record)   102 degrees
    Record lowest, January 1994 (39-year record)   21 degrees
    Normal heating degree days (30-year record)   4,665
    Normal cooling degree days (30-year record)   1,005
Precipitation
    Normal (30-year record)   41.49 inches
    Mean annual snowfall (30-year record)   25.7 inches
    Total precipitation, 1999   34.11 inches
    Mean number of days precipitation (30-year record)   139.7
    Mean number of days thunderstorms (30-year record)   40

Relative Humidity (30-Year Record)

1 a.m.	73 percent
7 a.m.	77 percent
1 p.m.	65 percent
7 p.m.	63 percent

Source: U.S. Department of Commerce, National Climatic Data Center, Local Climatological Data (1999). Station of record: Huntington, West Virginia.

Public School District Enrollments and Expenditures, 1998 to 1999

	Enrollment	Expenditures per Pupil	Pupil-to-Teacher Ratio
Ashland Independent	3,612	5,670	16.6
Boyd County	3,733	6,238	15.7
Fairview Independent	703	5,297	19.0
Greenup County	3,593	5,653	17.2
Raceland Independent	991	4,881	18.4
Russell Independent	2,278	5,019	18.7
Russell Independent	2,278	5,019	18.7

Source: Kentucky Department of Education, Office of Curriculum, Assessment and Accountability.

Nonpublic School Enrollments, 1999 to 2000

Number of Schools	Total Enrollment
7	920

Source: Kentucky Schools Directory, 1999–2000, Kentucky Department of Education.

Boyd and Greenup Counties Statistical Summary

Population, 1999	
Boyd and Greenup Counties	85,575
Labor market area	422,071
Business Cost	
Boyd and Greenup Counties per capita income	$21,687
Labor cost	90.8
Energy cost	65.8
Median household	$32,239
Median home price	$60,000
Kentucky has the eighth lowest overall business cost in the nation.	
Value-Added per Dollar of Production Wage, 1999	
Kentucky	$6.16
United States	$5.41
Kentucky has the eighth highest value-added per dollar of production wages in manufacturing (14% higher than the United States).	
Total Available Labor, 1999	
Boyd and Greenup Counties	17,475
Labor market area	78,583
Industrial Electric Cost per KWH, 1999	
Kentucky	$0.0299
United States	$0.0443
Kentucky is the fourth lowest cost state for industrial power.	
Unemployment Rate, 2000	
Boyd and Greenup Counties	5.1
Labor market area	6.5
United States	4.0
Average Weekly Wage, 1998	
Boyd and Greenup Counties	$543
Labor market area	$377
United States	$851

Boyd and Greenup Counties—Workforce

Total Available Labor, 1999

Unemployed	Potential Labor	Supply	Future Labor	Underemployed
78,583	13,465	10,032	55,086	31,349
17,475	2,602	1,882	12,991	6,019

Source: U.S. Department of Labor, Bureau of Labor Statistics, Kentucky Cabinet for Economic Development.

Civilian Labor Force

	Boyd and Greenup Counties		Labor Market Area	
	Jan. 2000	Dec. 2000	Jan. 2000	Dec. 2000
Civilian labor force	39,645	39,624	83,460	182,887
Employed	37,636	37,999	171,531	172,981
Unemployed	2,008	1,625	11,927	9,906
Unemployment rate (%)	5.1	4.1	6.5	5.4

Source: U.S. Department of Labor, Bureau of Labor Statistics. Preliminary annual averages.

Unemployment Rate (%)

Year	Boyd and Greenup Counties	Labor Market Area	Kentucky	United States
1996	6.9	7.9	5.6	5.4
1997	7.2	7.8	5.4	4.9
1998	6.2	7.3	4.6	4.5
1999	6.6	7.4	4.5	4.2
2000	5.1	6.5	3.9	4.0

Source: U.S. Department of Labor, Bureau of Labor Statistics. Year 2000 data are preliminary annual averages.

Average Weekly Wage ($), 1998

	Boyd and Greenup Counties	Kentucky	United States	Ohio
All industries	543	512	610	579
Mining and quarrying	N/A	808	1,000	813
Contract construction	486	543	641	650
Manufacturing	948	666	770	801
Transportation and utilities	697	686	756	698
Wholesale and retail trade	301	357	434	409
Finance, insurance, and real estate	547	652	935	736
Services	537	462	577	510
State and local government	N/A	494	598	586

	Indiana	Illinois	Tennessee	Virginia
All industries	560	668	546	595
Mining and quarrying	883	910	896	799
Contract construction	642	804	585	567
Manufacturing	772	816	641	670

	Indiana	Illinois	Tennessee	Virginia
Transportation and utilities	662	798	674	842
Wholesale and retail trade	371	479	413	416
Finance, insurance, and real estate	686	1,023	757	815
Services	476	608	521	628
State and local government	529	638	511	551

Source: U.S. Department of Labor, Bureau of Labor Statistics.

Commuting Patterns

	Boyd County Residents	Percent
Working and residing in the county	15,277	77.4
Commuting out of the county	4,449	22.6
Total residents	19,726	100.0
County employees	15,277	54.8
Commuting into the county	12,583	45.2
Total employees	27,860	100.0

Source: U.S. Department of Commerce, Bureau of the Census.

Boyd and Greenup Counties—Business and Industry

Summary of Recent Locations and Expansions, 1998 to Present

	Companies	Jobs	Investment
Manufacturing location	4	280	$22,710,000
Manufacturing expansion	14	50	$7,524,620
Supportive/service location	4	1,825	$14,530,000
Supportive/service expansion	3	653	$14,260,000

Source: Kentucky Cabinet for Economic Development. Employment by Major Industry by Place of Work, 1998.

Employment by Major Industry by Place of Work

	Boyd and Greenup Counties		Labor Market Area	
	Employment	Percent	Employment	Percent
All industries	36,206	100.0	144,236	100.0
Agriculture and forestry	180	0.5	N/A	N/A
Fishing mining and quarrying	N/A	N/A	N/A	N/A
Contract construction	1,829	5.1	6,853	4.8
Manufacturing	6,116	16.9	20,422	14.2
Transportation and utilities	2,042	5.6	N/A	N/A
Wholesale trade	1,660	4.6	N/A	N/A
Retail trade	8,435	23.3	33,255	23.1
Finance, insurance, and real estate	1,215	3.4	4,927	3.4
Services	9,184	25.4	38,456	26.7
State and local government	N/A	N/A	N/A	N/A
Other	N/A	N/A	N/A	N/A

Source: U.S. Department of Labor, Bureau of Labor Statistics.

Major Manufacturers

Firm	Product(s)	Employees	Year Established
Ashland			
AEI Resources, Inc.	Underground and surface coal mining	70	1984
AK Steel Corp.	Coke plant	383	1921
AK Steel Corp.	Flat rolled carbon steel	1,600	1921
Ashland Fabricating and Welding	Steel fabricating, arc and gas welding, and grinding; drilling, boring, cutting, and honing; and lathe and mill work	30	1954
Ashland Office Supply	Offset, letterpress, and screen printing; typesetting; and saddle stitch, perfect, and plastic binding	87	1957
Ashland Publishing Co.	Newspaper publishing	100	1921
Columbus Show Case Co.	Hardware fixtures and display showcases	64	1944
CONTECH Construction	Corrugated steel culvert pipe products	20	1966
Corbin, Ltd.	Men's and women's clothing—coats, jackets, skirts, blouses, shirts, suits, trousers, and shorts	400	1957
Gallaher's, Inc.	Commercial offset and letterpress printing; computer typesetting; and glue, saddle stitch, side and spiral wire, and perfect and plastic binding	35	1975
Heckett MultiServ	Crushed slag	50	1983
Hyland Co.	Pet food	20	1983
Kentucky Electric	Steel flat bars	400	1965
Marathon Ashland Petroleum, LLC	Research and development Laboratory	57	N/A
Pennco, Inc.	Glass and aluminum windows and patio doors	120	1956
R P M, Inc.	Industrial pump repairing and replacement parts	50	1992

Firm	Product(s)	Employees	Year Established
Riggs Machine and Fabricating	Machine shop: CNC and general fabricating machining; valve repairing; welding; mill and lathe work; and sheet plate, ornamental, and structural metal fabricating	57	1981
US Brick/Kline Plt.	Clay bricks	30	1926
Flatwoods			
Service Office Supplies	Offset and letterpress printing; typesetting; and glue, perfect, spiral, and side and saddle stitch binding	20	1982
Russell			
Raceland Car Shop	Freight cars and components	400	1929

Source: Kentucky Cabinet for Economic Development in cooperation with Harris InfoSource.

Boyd and Greenup Counties—Education and Training

Colleges and Universities Within 60 Miles of Ashland

Miles	Institution	Location	Enrollment (Fall 1997)
—	Ashland Community College	Ashland	2,271
5	Ohio University	Ironton	2,368
12	Marshall University	Huntington	11,066
18	Kentucky Christian College	Grayson	547
26	Shawnee State University	Portsmouth	3,505
47	Morehead State University	Morehead	8,208
55	West Virginia State College	Institute	4,545
55	Prestonsburg Community	Prestonburg	2,573
	Total Enrollments		**35,083**

Source: Kentucky Cabinet for Economic Development.

Kentucky Technical Schools Within 60 Miles of Ashland Enrollment (1997–1998)

Miles	Institution	Location	Sec	P/S	Total
—	Ashland Technical College	Ashland	0	670	670
—	Boyd County High Vocational School	Ashland	489	0	489
13	Greenup Co. ATC	Greenup	620	0	620
30	Carter County Vocational School	Olive Hill	170	0	170
38	Foster Mead Vocational Education Center	Vanceburg	215	0	215
41	Martin Co. ATC	Inez	45	0	245
45	Mayo Technical College	Paintsville	95	861	956
47	Rowan Co. Technical College	Morehead	99	417	516
5	Russell ATC	Russell	470	0	470
51	Morgan Co. ATC	West Liberty	221	0	221
	Total Enrollments		**2,624**	**1,948**	**4,572**

Source: Kentucky Cabinet for Workforce Development, Kentucky Community and Technical College System.

Training Resources

The Bluegrass State Skills Corporation (BSSC) was established in 1984 by the General Assembly of the Commonwealth of Kentucky as an independent, de jure corporation to stimulate economic development through customized business and industry specific skills training programs. The BSSC works with businesses, industries, and Kentucky's educational institutions to establish programs of skills training. The BSSC is attached to the Kentucky Cabinet for Economic Development for administrative purposes in recognition of the relationship between economic development and skills training efforts. The BSSC is comprised of two economic development tools: matching grants and recently authorized Skills Training Investment Tax Credit. The BSSC grant program is available to new, expanding and existing business and industry. Eligible training activities include pre-employment skills training and assessment, entry-level skills upgrade and occupational upgrade training; train-the-trainer travel, and capacity building. The Skills Training Investment Credit Act provides credits to existing businesses for skills upgrade training.

Information on other customized training, assessment services, and adult education services can be obtained by contacting the local economic development agency.

Bibliography

A mission statement from a Visiting Nurse Association. (February 6, 2003). Retrieved from http://www.users.cis.net/vna/mission.html

A U.S. Federal Government mission statement. (July 29, 2002). Retrieved from http://aspe.hhs.gov/hhsplan/

Academic Resource Center with time-management links. (March 10, 2002). Retrieved from http://www.arc.sbc.edu/timelinks.html

Agency for Healthcare Research and Quality. (May 5, 2002). Retrieved from http://www.ahcpr.gov

American Academy of Nurse Practitioners. (February 24, 2002). Contracting. Retrieved from http://www.aanp.org

American Academy of Nurse Practitioners. (February 24, 2002). Retrieved from http://www.aanp.org

American Academy of Nurse Practitioners. (February 24, 2002). Scope of practice and standards of practice. Retrieved from http://www.aanp.org

American College of Nurse Practitioners. (February 24, 2002). Direct Medicare reimbursement for nurse practitioners. Retrieved from http://www.nurse.org/acnp/medicare/

American College of Nurse Practitioners. (February 24, 2002). Retrieved from http://www.nurse.org.org/acnp

American Express Company. (February 18, 2002). American Express small business exchange: Creating an effective business plan. Retrieved from http://www.americanexpress.com/smallbusiness

American Nurses Association Safety and Quality Organization Links. (February 24, 2002). Retrieved from http://nursingworld.org/quality/links.htm

American Nurses Association. (1999). *Nursing quality indicators: Guide for implementation*. Washington, DC: American Nurses Association.

American Nurses Association. (2000). *Nursing quality indicators beyond acute care: Measurement instruments*. Washington, DC: American Nurses Association.

American Nurses Association. (February 24, 2002). Retrieved from http://www.nursingworld.org

Arcangelo, V., Fitzgerald, M., Carroll, D., & Plumb, J. D. (1996). Collaborative care between nurse practitioners and primary care physicians. *Primary Care: Clinics in Office Practice, 23*, 103–113.

Atlas Business Solutions. (April 12, 2002). Ultimate business planner. Retrieved from http://www.bptools.com/

Bain Publications. Management Tools. (April 12, 2002). Retrieved from http://www.bain.com/bainweb/expertise/tools/overview.asp

Ball, M. (Ed.). (2000). *Nursing informatics: Where caring and technology meet* (3rd ed.). New York: Springer-Verlag.

Bogart, J. B. (Ed.). (1998). *Legal nurse consulting principles and practice.* Boca Raton, FL: CRC Press.

Brache, A., & Freedman, M. (1999). Is our vision any good? *Journal of Business Strategy, 20,* 10–12.

Buppert, C. (1999). *Nurse practitioner's business practice & legal guide.* Gaithersberg, MD: Aspen Publishers.

Buppert, C. (2000). *The primary care provider's guide to compensation and quality* (1st ed.). Gaithersburg, MD: Aspen, Inc.

Buppert, C. (2001). Employee or independent contractor: What's the difference? *The Green Sheet, 3*(11): Law Office of Carolyn Buppert, Annapolis, MD.

Buppert, C. (2001). How can I start my own nonprofit clinic? *Medscape Nurses, 3*(2). Retrieved May 12, 2002 from http://www.medscape.com/viewarticle/413366

Buppert, C. (2001). How NPs can increase profits from their practices? *The Green Sheet, 13*(10): Law Office of Carolyn Buppert, Annapolis, MD.

Buppert, C. (2001). What information can you give me about independent NP practices? *Medscape Nurse, 3.* Retrieved May 12, 2002 from http://www.medscape.com/viewarticle/413411

Buppert, C. (2002). What do I need to consider before starting an NP practice? *Medscape Nurse, 4.* Retrieved May 12, 2002 from http://www.medscape.com/viewarticle/429842

Canadian Bankers Association. (2001). Getting started in small business. Retrieved February 3, 2002, from http://www.cba/eng/Tools/Brochures/tools_small.cfm?pg=3

Carpentino, L. J. (1998). Redefining the gold standard of health care AKA medical care. *Nursing Forum, 33,* 3–4.

Center for Entrepreneurial Studies and Development. (February 6, 2003). Process management. Retrieved from http://www.cesd.wvu.edu

Certification Boards for Nurse Practitioner. (February 6, 2003.). Retrieved from http://www.npcentral.net/resources/certification

Christensen, C. M., Bohmer, R., & Kenagy, J. (2000). Will disruptive innovations cure health care? *Harvard Business Review, 78,* 102–112.

CLIA Program Clinical Laboratory Improvement Amendment. (February 6, 2003). Retrieved from http://www.cms.hhs.gov.clia

Coiera, E. (1997). *Guide to medical informatics, the Internet, and telemedicine* (1st ed.). New York: Oxford University Press.

Collins, J. C., & Porras, J. I. (1997). *Built to last: Successful habits of visionary companies.* New York: HarperBusiness.

Czar, P., Mascara, C., Hebda, T. L., & Mascara, C. M. (2001). *Handbook of informatics for nurses and health care professionals* (2nd ed.). Upper Saddle River, NJ: Prentice-Hall.

Devore, N.E. (1999). Telephone triage: A challenge for practicing midwives. *Journal of Nurse-Midwifery, 44*, 471–479.

Dienemann, J. (Ed.). (1992). *Continuous quality improvement in nursing.* Washington, D.C.: American Nurses Association.

Drucker, P. (1974). *Management: Tasks, responsibilities, politics.* New York: Harper & Row.

Electronic Journal of Radical Organization Theory (February 1, 2003). Retrieved from http://www.mngt.waikato.ac.nz/research/ejrot/

eMedicine Journal, and eMedicine World Medical Library. (February 12, 2002). Instant access to the minds of medicine. Retrieved from http://www.emedicine.com

Entrepreneur Magazine. (February 12, 2002). Entrepreneur Magazine's small business square. Retrieved from http://www.entrepreneurmag.com

Entrepreneur. (2002). Solutions for growing businesses. Retrieved from http://www.entrepreneur.com/Your_Business/YB_SegArticle/0,4621.287323—1-00.html

Fankhauser, J. (1982). *From a chicken to an eagle.* Farmingdale, NY: Coleman Graphics.

Fisher, R., & Ury, W. (1991). *Getting to yes* (2nd ed.). New York: Penguin Books.

Franklin Electronic Publishers (February 21, 2002). Franklin electronic publisher's medical products. Retrieved from http://www.franklin.com

Gegor, C. (1997). Do's and don'ts of clinical practice guidelines. *Quickening, 28*(3), 13–14.

Golanty, E. (1995–2002). Physician's guide to the Internet. (February 28, 2002). Retrieved from http://www.webcom.com/pgi/

Gordon, M. Business vision quest: Guidelines for writing your business vision statement. (February 21, 2002). Retrieved from http://www.mollygordon.com

Guidi, T. U., & Gruber, J. (2001). Marketing for the oncology practice. *Oncology Issues, 16*(2), 26–28.

Hamric, A. B., Spross, J. A., & Hanson, C. M. (2000). *Advanced practice nursing: An integrative approach* (2nd ed.). Philadelphia: Saunders.

Hannah, K. J., Ball, M. J., & Edwards, M. J. A. (1999). *Introduction to nursing informatics* (2nd ed.). New York: Springer-Verlag.

Harvard Business Review. (February 10, 2002). Retrieved from http://hbsp.harvard.edu/products/hbr/

Hawkins, J., & Thibodeau, J. (1996). *The advanced practice nurse current issues* (4th ed.). New York: Tiresias Press.

Health Care Financing Administration. (1997). Documentation guidelines for evaluation and management services. Retrieved February 28, 2002 from http://www.hcfa.gov/medicare/mcarpti.htm

Heitz, T. M., & VanDinter, M. (2000). Developing collaborative practice agreements. *Journal of Pediatric Health Care, 14*, 200–203.

Henricks, M. (1999). *Business plans made easy.* Irvine, CA: Entrepreneur Media.

Hersey, P., Blanchard, K. H., & Johnson, D. E. (1996). *Management of organizational behavior: Utilizing human resources* (7th ed.). Upper Saddle River, NJ: Prentice-Hall.

Hickey, J. V., Ouimette, R. M., & Venegoni, S. L. (1996). *Advanced practice nursing: Changing roles and clinical applications.* Philadelphia: Lippincott.

Hill, C. W. L., & Jones, G. R. (2001). *Strategic management: An integrated approach* (5th ed., Rev. ed.). Boston: Houghton Mifflin Company.

How to draft a mission statement. Retrieved February 8, 2003 from http://www.acnm.org

Huber, D. (2000). *Leadership and nursing care management* (2nd ed.). Philadelphia: W. B. Saunders.

Hunsicker, F., & Langford, B. An integrated view of the relationship between the organization and its environment. Retrieved February 28, 2002 from http://www.westga.edu:80/~bquest/1996/model.html

Hurdle. (2001). Yahoo small business planning guide. Retrieved February 2, 2002, from http://smallbusiness.yahoo.com/start_a_new_business/business_planning/business_planning_quck.html

Institute for Quality Improvement. Retrieved February 20, 2002 from http://www.aaahciqi.org

Institute of Medicine (1990). *Medicine: A strategy for quality assurance* (Vol. I). Washington, D.C.: National Academy Press.

Internet Journal of Advanced Nursing Practice. (1997). Defining scope of practice. Retrieved May 10, 2002 from http://www.ispub.com/journals/IJANP/Vol1N2/Scope.htm

Jacob, J. A. (2002). Keys to a successful practice. *America Medical News, 45*(12).

JCAHO facts about ORYX and performance measurement requirements for health care organizations. Retrieved February 6, 2003 from http://www.jcaho.org/pms/index.htm

Kleinpell, R. M. (1998). *Practice issues for the acute care nurse practitioner.* New York: Springer Publishing.

Kozier, B., Erb, G., & Blais, K. (1997). *Professional nursing practice: Concepts and perspectives* (3rd ed.). New York: Addison-Wesley.

Kritek, P. B. (1994). *Negotiating at an uneven table.* San Francisco: Jossey-Bass Publishers.

Kuskey, K. (1996). Standards for vision statements: A discussion thread. Retrieved January 23, 2002, from Electronic Discussion on Group Facilitation Web Site: http://www.albany.edu/cpr/gf/resources/Vision.html

Levine, J., Baroudi, C., & Levine, M. (2002). The Internet for dummies (5th ed.). New York: IDG Books Worldwide.

Lewis-Ford, B. (1993). Management techniques: Coping with difficult people. *Nursing Management, 24*(3), 36–38.

Lusky, P. (1998). *Slam the door on employee lawsuits: Keep your business out of court.* Franklin Lakes, NJ: Career Press.

Marquis, B.L., & Huston, C.J. (1996). *Leadership roles and management functions in nursing: Theory and application.* Philadelphia: Lippincott.

Mathews, R., & Wacker, W. (2002). Deviants, Inc. *Fast Company, 56,* 70–80.

McKeever, M. (1999). *How to write a business plan* (5th ed.). Berkley, CA: Nolo.

McLaughlin, C. P., & Kaluzny, A. D. (Eds.). (1999). *Continuous quality improvement in health care.* Gaithersburg, MD: Aspen Publishers, Inc.

Medscape Portals, Inc. (2002). Medscape. Retrieved February 10, 2002 from http://www.medscape.com/px/urlinfo

Microsoft® Encarta® Online Encyclopedia 2001. Advertising. Retrieved February 28, 2002 from http://encarta.msn.com ©1997–2000 Microsoft Corporation.

Milio, N. (2002). A new leadership role for nursing in a globalized world. *Topics in Advanced Practice Nursing eJournal, 2.* Retrieved February 28, 2002 from http://www.medscape.com/viewarticle/421474

National Committee for Quality Assurance. (n.d.). Retrieved May 10, 2002 from http://www.ncqa.org

National Safety Council. Retrieved May 10, 2002 from http://www.nsc.org

Neale, J. (1999). Nurse practitioners and physicians: A collaborative practice. *Clinical Nurse Specialist, 13,* 252–258.

Norris, J. (2002). Nursing informatics. Retrieved March 18, 2002 from http://www.nursinginformatics.net

Norris, J. R. (2002). The nursing theory page. Retrieved February 28, 2002 from http://www.ualberta.ca/-jrnorris/nt/theory.html

Norsen, L., Opladen, J., & Quinn, J. (1995). Collaborative practice. *Critical Care Clinics of North America, 7,* 43–52.

North Mississippi Health Services (2002). Patient survey of health care of clinic. Family medicine clinic of Oxford. Oxford, Mississippi.

NP Central Gateway. Retrieved February 10, 2002, from http://www.nurse.net/

NP Central. (2001). NP Central: Information for and about nurse practitioners. Retrieved February 10, 2002 from http://www.nurse.net/index.shtml/

Nurse Practitioner Profession. (n.d.). Retrieved May 12, 2002 from http://www .nlm. nih.gov/medlineplus/ency/articl/001934.htm

Nurse Practitioner Support Services (October 19, 2001). The search resource for nurse practitioners and clinics. Retrieved January 28, 2002 from http://npclin-ics.com

Nurses Station. (n.d.). Nursing and healthcare directories: The Nursefriendly nurse practitioners. Advanced Practice Nursing. Retrieved May 12, 2002 from http:// www.nursefriendly.com/np

OASIS Data Sets and Forms—Health Care Financing Administration. (n.d.). Retrieved March 18, 2002 from http://www.hcfa.gov/medicaid/oasis/ oasisdat.htm

On-Line Journal of Nursing Informatics. (1999). Nursing Informatics of International Medical Informatics Association. Retrieved February 12, 2002 from http://cac.psu.edu/~dxm12/OJNI.html

Orman, Levent V. A Model Management Approach to Business Process Reengineering. Retrieved January 28, 2002 from http://hsb.baylor.edu/ramsower/acis/papers/orman.htm

Pearson, L. (2002). Fourteenth annual legislative update: How each state stands on legislative issues affecting advanced nursing practice. *Nurse Practitioner, 27,* 10–22.

Pinson, L., & Jinnett, J. (1999). *Anatomy of a business plan.* Chicago: Dearborn.

Radtke, J. M. (1998). How to write a mission statement. Retrieved May 12, 2002 from http://www.tgci.com/publications/98fall/MissionStatement.html

Rehm, S., & Kraft, S. (1998). How to select a computer system for a family physician's office. Retrieved February 12, 2002 from http://www.aafp.org/fpnet/guide/

Rieder, M. (1999). Effective practice marketing. *Physicians Financial News, 17*(11), 14–18.

Schneider, P. (2002). Creating your mission statement for work and for life. Retrieved February 28, 2002 from Nursing Spectrum Career Fitness Online Web Site http://nsweb.nursingspectrum.com/cfforms/missionstatement.cfm

Sebas, M. B. (1994). Developing a collaborative practice agreement for the primary care setting. *Nurse Practitioner, 19*(3), 49–51.

Sheer, B. (2001). New horizons for nurse practitioners around the world. *Medscape Nurses, 3*(2). Retrieved May 10, 2002 from http://www.medscape.com/viewarticle/408428

Sherwood, G. D. (1997). Nurse practitioner descriptions for primary care centers: Opportunities for ownership. *Journal of the American Academy of Nurse Practitioners, 9,* 462–469.

Shortliffe, E. (Ed.). (2000). *Medical Informatics: Computer Applications in Health Care and Biomedicine (Health Informatics)* (2nd ed.). New York: Springer-Verlag.

Simms, L. M., Price, S. A., & Ervin, N. E. (2000). *The professional practice of nursing administration* (3rd ed.). Albany: Delmar.

Small Business Development Center. (2001). Small business administration. Retrieved February 2, 2002, from http://www.sbaonling.sba.gov

Smithing, R. (2002). NP Central: Information for and about nurse practitioners. Retrieved February 28, 2000 from http://www.nurse.net

Society for Risk Analysis. Retrieved January 28, 2002 from http://www.sra.org

Sox, H. C. (2000). Independent primary care practice by nurse practitioners. JAMA. Retrieved May 12, 2002 from http://jama.ama-assn.org/issues/v283nl/ffull/jed90087.html

Stangler, R. S. (2001). Towards global health: the informatic route to knowledge. *MedscapeTechMed*, *1*(2). Retrieved March 18, 2002 from http://www.medscape.com/viewartilce/415046

Stress-management links. (n.d.). Retrieved February 10, 2002 from http://imt.net/~randolfi/StressLinks.html

The American Health Quality Association. Retrieved January 24, 2002 from http://www.ahqa.org

The Ohio Center for Critical Thinking Instruction. Retrieved February 12, 2002 from http://www.acorn.net/lists-ht/occti.html

The Strategic Planning Process for HealthCare Organizations. (n.d.). Retrieved March 10, 2002 from http://healthinfo.montana.edu/mtahec/stratpln.html

Thede, L. (1992). Data Base Systems. In J. Arnold & G. Pearson (Eds.), *Computers in nursing practice, education, and research*. New York: National League for Nursing.

U.S. Department of Justice: Drug Enforcement Administration (2002). Drug registration: DEA. Retrieved March 3, 2002, from http://www.DEAdiversion.usdoj.gov

Walter, R. (2000). *The secret guide to computers: This is the best computer book.* (26th ed.). New York: Russell Walter Publishing.

Weisman, C. S., Grason, H. A., & Strobino, D. S. (2001). Quality management in public and community health: Examples from women's health. *Quality Management in Health Care*, *10*, 54–64.

Whythe, E. G., & Blair, J. D. (1995). Strategic planning for health care provider organizations. In L. F. Wolfer (Ed.), *Health care administration: Principles, practices, structure, and delivery* (2nd ed.). Gaithersburg, MD: Aspen.

Wold, J. L., Stanhope, M., & Lancaster, M. (2002). *Community Health Nursing* (5th ed.). St. Louis, MO: Mosby.

Zaumeyer, C. (n.d.). The NP as entrepreneur: How to establish and operate an independent practice. Retrieved May 12, 2002 from http://www.independentnp.com

Index

CPSIA information can be obtained at www.ICGtesting.com
Printed in the USA
BVOW02*0120080114

341185BV00007B/287/A